MEDICAL BILLING

THE BOTTOM LINE

REVISED EDITION

INCLUDES

UNDERSTANDING MEDICAL BILLING

CLAUDIA A. YALDEN

Medical Billing – The Bottom Line

MEDICAL BILLING: THE BOTTOM LINE
Copyright © 1997 by Claudia A. Yalden
Revised 1999

This publication is designed to provide accurate and authoritative information with regard to the subject matter covered. It is sold with the understanding that the author is not engaged in rendering legal, accounting, or other professional advice. If legal or other expert assistance is required, the services of a qualified professional person should be sought.

- *From a Declaration of Principles jointly adapted by a Committee of the American Bar Association and a Committee of Publishers and Associations.*

To order additional copies call 1-800-221-0488

Cover design and Typesetting by Claudia A. Yalden

CAY Medical Management, Inc.
Post Office Box 958
Bridgeton, North Carolina 28519-0958

603-465-6062/ fax 603-465-9610

ISBN: 0-7392-0361-4
Library of Congress Catalog Card Number: 99-93511

Printed in the USA by

MORRIS PUBLISHING
3212 East Highway 30 • Kearney, NE 68847 • 1-800-650-7888

This book is dedicated to my wonderful father

**Captain Pierre R. Becker, USNR Retired
And
Kings Point Class of '42**

Watching my Dad and the effort he devoted to his own book and CD Rom -

*"Personal History
Of Cadets, Midshipman and Officers
In the US Merchant Marine Cadet Corps And
US Merchant Marine Academy
Graduates Of 1942"*

encouraged me to revise -

Medical Billing The Bottom Line

Without his inspiration and support I could never have finished.

I love you dad.

April 20, 1922 – August 31, 1998

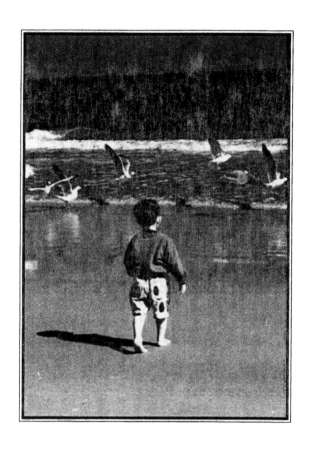

You Cannot Discover New Oceans

Unless You Have The Courage

To Lose Sight Of The Shore

— *Successories,* 1996

CHAPTER 1
THE BOTTOM LINE   15

CHAPTER 2
OBTAINING FINANCIAL HELP   21

CHAPTER 3
SETTING UP YOUR HOME OFFICE   25

CHAPTER 4
THE BUSINESS PLAN   29

CHAPTER 5
WRITING A BUSINESS PLAN   31

CHAPTER 6
GETTING STARTED AND NETWORKING   39

CHAPTER 7
SUPERBILLS AND CLAIM FORMS   43

CHAPTER 8
REFERENCE BOOKS   45

CHAPTER 9
WHAT DOCTORS WANT TO HEAR   53

CHAPTER 10
PRICING YOUR SERVICES   59

CHAPTER 11
Marketing Strategies   69

CHAPTER 12
NEWSPAPERS
FOLLOWING THE HELP WANTED ADS   75

CHAPTER 13
DIRECT MARKETING   81

CHAPTER 14
DIRECT MAIL   85

CHAPTER 15
LETTERS, FLYERS AND OTHER TECHNIQUES   97

CHAPTER 16
PACKETS AND WHAT TO INCLUDE   117

CHAPTER 17
THE PRESENTATION   131

CHAPTER 18
CONTRACTS, AGREEMENTS, & FORM   139

CHAPTER 19
SOFTWARE & THEIR COST   151

CHAPTER 20
COMMON QUESTIONS & ANSWERS   157

CHAPTER 21
UNDERSTANDING MEDICAL BILLING   163

CHAPTER 22
MEDICAL TERMINOLOGY   165

CHAPTER 23
INTRODUCTION INTO MEDICAL BILLING 187

CHAPTER 24
LEGAL CONSIDERATION 191

CHAPTER 25
LIFE CYCLE OF AN INSURANCE CLAIM 205

CHAPTER 26
THE CPT FORMAT 215

CHAPTER 27
UNDERSTANDING HCPC CODES 225

CHAPTER 28
ICD-9CM DIAGNOSTIC CODING 241

CHAPTER 29
V CODES 247

CHAPTER 30
E CODES 249

CHAPTER 31
M CODES 251

CHAPTER 32
FORMS 253

CHAPTER 33
WEB ADDRESS PAGE 261

INTRODUCTION

MY MESSAGE TO YOU . . .

Many people and forces helped me make this book possible. It was designed and written to help the many people who are interested in a home based medical or dental billing business and don't know where to begin. I was there once and found out there is no ready reference books available.

This book will tell you that everything is possible and I thank my parents, *Mildred and Pierre Becker*, who made me possible. The first page and the last pages could not have been written without the loving support and tolerance of my special husband, Robert, and my determination to watch my grandson Patrick grow up. They were literally by my side throughout the process. And special thanks for the ongoing encouragement of my two sons Robert and Jeffrey and my daughter Christin who encouraged me from the beginning and told me I could do it.

There are no words to thank my colleague and friend Jo-Anne Sheehan whose encouragement and professional ideas helped me finish and put my ideas into writing. It was through this book that Jo-Anne became my "very dear friend." And a special thanks to Beverly, Lois, Bruce, Sally and all my Prodigy friends for all their inspiration, ideas, help and most of all their support.

As you travel through this book learning how you too can be an entrepreneur and fulfill your dreams you will see where I made mistakes which cost me thousands of dollars.   After many questions and problems I decided that a book needed to be written to help people who, like me, wanted to get into this business without spending a lot of money.

I started my medical billing business to get out of the rat race of commuting to Boston and to be with my grandson, Patrick.   I always wanted to be an entrepreneur and enjoyed medical billing when I was living in Port Jefferson, New York.   I was away from billing for over ten years but felt having a background working in the Child Development Unit at Children's Hospital in Boston with Dr. Terry B. Brazelton would be an asset and a credit that would allow me to easily get started.   I never realized how changes and time affected billing.   Just as television, the greatest invention of its time was sold in black and white and later went on to be sold in color, so is the medical billing business.   Claims were once submitted.   Doctors were paid.   Secondary insurance was filed.   There was no Capitation, adjustments, write-offs, Managed Care and there was no medigap.

This book is designed to give you the knowledge to get started in the electronic medical billing industry; ideas on financial help; equipment needed; and office operation suggestions.   Through my experience of failures and successes, and the knowledge I've gained from so many people, I have decided to share with you ideas on marketing strategies.   For the new entrepreneur I introduce books and organizations.   You'll read some true experience and common questions and answers that many people need to know.

This books is written as a layman's manual, giving ideas of the basic "*nuts and bolts*" of the business and hopefully assisting you in your decision - is this right for me? My desire is for you to gain insight toward financial benefit of a business like this and how to price your services. Last but not least, I refer to areas concerning medical software and understanding medical billing. My hope is for you to understand what is needed, the pitfalls you may face, and how to succeed from the beginning.

Although all your questions will not be answered, it is the beginning of learning the business. There are still many experts in the field who may be able to help you. However, if you cannot find the answer to your questions, please feel free to contact me and I will assist you in finding someone who can help. I needed the support and used it. My new goal is to help support you.

Good luck in your business,

and remember . . .

don't give up!

Claudia A. Yalden
New Hampshire

July 1999

CHAPTER 1

THE BOTTOM LINE

Many people think about going into a home based business and become the entrepreneur of the 21st century, and become independently wealthy or maybe comfortable. They want to pay off their bills, send their children to college, drive the car of their dreams, vacation in the sun, or have a bank account where you don't have to balance it. Or maybe you just want some extra income to supplement what you already have, or possibly you want something to fall back on in retirement. Whatever your reasons, you have decided you want to investigate a Medical or Dental home-based electronic billing business.

Although electronic claims submission is growing . . . it still has a long way to go. The market is huge.

Each year the percentage of electronic claims being filed is growing. Although it is encouraging, let's look at the other side of this coin. Each year big powerful Health Maintenance Organizations (HMO) and Preferred Provider Organizations (PPO) are buying out more and more medical practices. That could possibility mean they will have their own capability to file their claims electronically and have no need for you, or they could realize the benefits of outsourcing and you may be able to land the account. The bottom line I would like to stress to you is that this business will take time.

You will not get rich quickly, and if that is the reason you are contemplating going into this business, then I suggest you save your money. This business will take time, perseverance, persistence and education. You need to market and you need to be determined not to quit, not to get discouraged and you need to follow a marketing plan faithfully. Only when you can commit to that will you be able to make money and know that this business will work, but "*it will take time*."

Some of the responsibilities you will face as you proceed in this business are:

✓ Gaining knowledge of medical terminology.

✓ Posting charges, payments and adjustments to the patient's accounts.

✓ Applying knowledge of filing rules and regulations for major insurance programs and Medicaid programs.

✓ Coding accurately all procedures and diagnosis (if applicable).

✓ Prepare and file for all types of medical and disability claims.

✓ Review insurance payments and copies of original claims to check the claim summaries and ensure proper payment of the claim.

✓ Prepare appeals for all underpaid claims.

✓ Re-bill all insurance claims not paid within 30 to 45 days.

✓ Inform health care providers of changes in insurance requirements.

✓ Maintain an audit system that ensures all required managed care pre-authorizations and treatment reports are obtained and conveyed to the authorizing agent prior to the patient receiving services (if applicable).

✓ Explain insurance benefits, policy requirements, and filing procedures to patients (if applicable).

So . . . if you're still contemplating going into the Medical or Dental Billing business I will share ideas and suggest a direction on how to market. There is an example of how to write a business plan and the importance of it.

When I began this business I thought that I should only target my market on the small town family doctors or narrow in on the specialties that were not part of an HMO, PPO. Years later my thoughts changed because even doctors that are part of an HMO or PPO are in need of your service. Doctor's in a big medical or dental center are in need of your service. There are some big opportunities out there and if you don't try and market them, someone else will. Ambulance companies and Durable Medical Equipment suppliers are great to target in on. Very few ambulance companies utilize electronic billing and all the advantages that go with it. Durable Medical Equipment is an entirely different kind of billing but they too have to submit claims for wheelchairs, walkers, crutches, ostomy supplies, etc. Don't overlook any opportunity.

Businesses fail because the majority of small business owners have a work mentality, not a business mentality.

In this business you will need both. You will continually need to educate yourself by joining organizations and reading everything available to keep abreast of the continuing healthcare changes. You need to contact your Medicare/Medicaid office in your state. Get on their mailing list and tell them you want to be notified of any seminars coming up. Call your Blue Cross/Blue Shield office. They too offer seminars. The best part of these seminars is that they are generally free. Check with the local hospitals for seminars they sponsor. Attend as many as you possibility can.

You can make money in this business but I cannot emphasize enough that –

"The name of the game is perseverance."

I have outlined the basics of getting started, marketing, obtaining software and pricing your services. After that, it is up to you.

There are organizations and networking groups available. You can find most of these on the Internet Bulletin Boards. I suggest using Yahoo or any of the other search engines available to do a search for Medical or Dental Billing information.

You will also be receiving updates from your software vendor or clearinghouse. Access the HCFA web site which has valuable information and constant updates. You will be providing electronic claim submission for physicians and other health care providers and you will be soaring to new heights in your development and career.

Your responsibilities as a medical claims specialist or billing service will include:

- Knowledge of medical terminology.

- Post charges, payments and adjustments to the patient's ledger.

- Abstract patient charts and ledgers for proper filing of insurance claims (if applicable).

- Apply knowledge of filing rules and regulations for major insurance programs and Medicaid programs.

- Code accurately all procedures and diagnosis (if applicable).

- Prepare accurately and file all types of medical and disability claims.

- Review insurance payments and copies of original claims to check the claim summaries and ensure proper payment of the claim.

- Prepare appeals for all underpaid claims.

- Re-bill all insurance claims not paid within 30 to 45 days.

- Inform health care providers and staff of changes in insurance requirements.

- Keep the practice's internal documents updated such as patient registration forms and charges.

- Update forms as required by changes in coding or insurance billing requirements.

- Maintain an audit system that ensures all required managed care pre-authorizations and treatment reports are obtained and conveyed to the authorizing agent **prior** to the patient receiving services (if applicable).

- Explain insurance benefits, policy requirements, and filing procedures to patients and sometimes physicians (if applicable).

CHAPTER 2

OBTAINING FINANCIAL HELP

There are many agencies willing to give grants. A lot of these grants do not have to be paid back.

You can obtain information on grants from the local library or on the Internet. A book worth reading on obtaining grants is **"The Action Guide to Government Grants, Loans, and Giveaways,"** by George Chelekis which is a comprehensive guide to getting millions of dollars in grants, loan guarantees, loans, and other financial help from federal and state government sources. It is well worth the investment or borrow the book from your local library.

The entire government grants and loan awards process has, in the past, gotten a bad rap from the media. It probably deserved it since not only were tax dollars wasted, but the projects funded just did not make sense. Government and private funding were being used for such things as a quick-cooked hamburger that cooks in less than 30 seconds with no smoke and no pre-heating of the grill. It's no wonder they received a bad rap!

There are certain guidelines, which need to be followed if you are to obtain a loan or grant.

They are:

- ✓ A financial statement which includes a balance sheet and profit and loss statement.

- ✓ A resume of management and brief history of the business.

- ✓ Loan proposal, outlining the use of proceeds of the loan and maturity needed.

- ✓ One year profit and loss projection.

For additional information, contact the **U. S. Small Business Administration** at **1-800-8-ASK-SBA** and ask for the number of your local SBA office.

You can also obtain information at any of the following sources:

- ➢ SBA District Offices

- ➢ Small Business Development Centers (SBDCs)

- ➢ Service Corps of Retired Executives (SCORE)

- ➢ Small Business Institutes (SBIs)

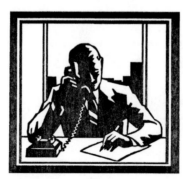

SBA offers small business loans of $100,000 or less. They guarantee up to 90% of the loan. You can generally get a response within 2 or 3 days. Interest rates cannot exceed SBA maximums and the length of time for repayment depends on your ability to:

✓ Repay.

✓ The use of the loan proceeds.

✓ And may not exceed 25 years for fixed assets or 10 years for all other uses.

You will need:

✓ A current business balance sheet

✓ A profit and loss statement

✓ Personal financial statement

✓ A list of collateral to be offered

SCORE is a 13,000 member volunteer program sponsored by the SBA. They offer management counseling and training for small businesses and to those considering going into business. They also offer pre-business workshops as well as a variety of other workshops nationwide to prospective small business entrepreneurs.

Among other things, they have training and educational programs, advisory services, publications, financial programs, and contract assistance. **SCORE** specializes in programs for women business owners, minorities, veterans, international trade, and rural development.

Money - While many software company's charge anywhere from $99 to $20,000, CAYMM has several options. Our most popular training package is our one-on-one hands on training package. Most people prefer the personalized attention from Claudia to ensure they get the individual attention they deserve. Our next training package is the $1499. package which is for someone who feels they have the medical billing knowledge already and needs to learn software and marketing. Our low end package which sells for $299 is designed for those with a limited budget and feel they have the motivation and desire for self-training.

Space - A billing center can be started in the corner of a room. The minimum requirement is a phone, computer system, and a work table. Appointments with physicians are conducted at their office.

Equipment - Computer, phone, fax/modem, copier, file cabinet, general office supplies (stapler, tape, etc.).

Time - Many billing center owners start by working part-time processing claims. Naturally, the more time you put into the business the faster the business will grow. One person could easily handle ten physicians, depending on their specialty.

Legal - Currently there are no known special licenses or certificates to operate a medical billing service; however it is always advisable to check with your town about a home-based business.

Marketing – Our marketing book guides you through the marketing process with plenty of sample pieces. You can spend as little or as much in marketing as your budget allows.

Commitment - You need motivation, persistence, and determination. If you have these – you're on your way!

Starting A Billing Service
Takes Motivation,
Determination, and Faith

CHAPTER 3

SETTING-UP YOUR HOME OFFICE

Your computer and software are your primary tools. Most software is for an IBM clone but there are a few companies who sell for MacIntosh as well. You will also need a printer, modem, and a dedicated phone line with an answering machine. Most computers come with a built-in fax/modem. If your computer does not have a built-in modem you will have to buy an external modem.

For furniture, looking in second hand office furniture stores will save you money and you can find almost anything you need to get started in your business.

Once you're in business a fax machine is a real asset. You would be amazed at how much work you can do via a fax. If your computer has a built-in fax/modem, that's great . . . except there are times when you need to fax information that is not on your computer. A built-in fax/modem is not always dependable either. I think technology has a long way to go before fax/modems will work properly.

I have had people ask me to fax information to them and when I did they answered the phone. When I explain that I am trying to fax I get "*Oh, I'm sorry. I'll turn on the fax, give me a minute.*" It is frustrating to the person who is faxing. I do not like to fax to anyone unless they have a dedicated fax telephone number.

Personally, a separate fax, apart from your computer, is your best bet. A separate fax will serve as an interim copy machine as well. There are hundreds of different fax machines on the market. When I started out I purchased a used thermal fax machine which ran for years. If your budget allows I recommend a plain paper fax machine because of quality in making copies and greater legibility in materials being faxed to you. Thermal fax paper will fade over a period of time. Prices are falling. Just remember you don't want to spend a lot of money at first.

KEEP IT SIMPLE, KEEP IT INEXPENSIVE.
AND, IF POSSIBLE
GO FOR A SEPARATE FAX MACHINE.

FILE CABINETS –

File cabinets are extremely useful. You will find that the more information you receive in the mail, the more information you will want to keep. Keeping organized and having the ability to readily access any information you will need will come in handy when you keep a good filing system. It also reduces stress when you know where to look for something. I have gone through the stress of not being organized, and we are all guilty of it, so I cannot stress enough the importance of being organized.

ROLODEX –

Using a rolodex! You will be amazed at how many numbers you will acquire even if you're only working with one account in the beginning. There are numbers you will use often and there are numbers you will only use once a year. Having numbers readily available saves you a lot of time when you need to order books, HCFA paper, supplies, etc. You will also start networking via the Internet or whatever on-line services you join and acquire new numbers. There will be contacts and people you will want to stay in touch with and a Rolodex is a good way to remain organized.

I feel many of us, myself especially, are guilty of scribbling phone numbers on small pieces of paper or stick-em's, only to be sorry later when the number is lost. Get in the habit of using a Rolodex and keep it right by your computer. There is software available for keeping phone numbers however I recommend using a Rolodex for immediate accessibility.

PLANNER –

There are many various yearly planners on the market today. I find it to be an essential tool and I always carry one. I use a Franklin Planner. It offers me the opportunity to prioritize my schedule and enables me to write a list of things to do. I write everything in my planner so there is always a record. When I'm near a phone, I always have my planner with me. Again, loose paper and stick-em's only become lost later on. If you don't want a planner in the beginning, use a notebook. The important key here is keeping everything together - even your mental notes.

It has been said that the most successful people are the most organized. Make your home office as organized and easy to maneuver around in as possible. It will make your life easier and your business will flow that much more readily.

BOOKKEEPING –

I recommend the Dome Simplified Weekly Bookkeeping Record for a weekly record of expenses and income. This will greatly assist you in tracking your business expenses and will make life easier in preparing your tax return.

Steps To Take

⇒ In order to succeed, if you have no prior experience – obtain the necessary training. In order to feel confident you will need a good training foundation which will be your key to success. If you don't have the money to invest in training you are short changing yourself.

⇒ Decide on what software you want to use.

⇒ Decide on a name for your business.

⇒ Call your local town hall and check zoning laws. If applicable you may need to apply for a business license.

⇒ Consult a lawyer regarding legal issues such whether to incorporate or register, etc.

⇒ Consult an accountant regarding tax and bookkeeping issues.

⇒ Write a business and marketing plan.

⇒ Decide where to set up your office.

⇒ Install a business phone and/or a dedicated fax line.

⇒ Open a business bank account.

⇒ Set up bookkeeping system (I started with the Dome Simplified Weekly Bookkeeping Record and graduated to Quick Books).

⇒ Design and print business cards and stationary.

⇒ Create marketing materials to send out.

⇒ Purchase necessary office equipment, supplies, file cabinets, etc. You will also need HCFA forms, envelopes, and paper.

⇒ Locate a clearinghouse and get the necessary paperwork before you begin to market.

⇒ Purchase the ICD-9 and CPT coding books along with any other reference books you desire.

⇒ If possible get on Medicare and Medicaid mailing lists. You may not be able to if you do not have a provider.

⇒ Subscribe to publications and join organizations

CHAPTER 4.

THE BUSINESS PLAN

Successful small business expansions and new job formations lead the way in creating new markets, innovations, and jobs. Most entrepreneurs are not adequately prepared to go into business. Although they have the desire, talent, and motivation . . . many have not taken the time to properly investigate and research the business they are interested in starting.

A business plan is very important. Many people, myself included, dive right into a business venture and don't bother with a business plan. Or they start a business and tell themselves they will write a business plan "*later.*" Only later never comes.

Let's determine why people go into business:

COMMON REASONS FOR STARTING A BUSINESS:

➢ Being your own boss
➢ Financial freedom
➢ Not working for others

DETERMINING WHAT IS THE RIGHT BUSINESS FOR YOU:

- ✓ What do you like to do with your time?
- ✓ What skills do you have? Have you developed those skills?
- ✓ What support from family and friends will you get?
- ✓ How much time are you ready to devote to the business?
- ✓ What skills do you have that are marketable?

AND THEN

- ✓ What finances will you need?
- ✓ Can you operate your business for approximately 1 year with little or no income?
- ✓ Is your idea practical, and will it fill a need?
- ✓ What is your competition?
- ✓ What is your advantage over an existing business?
- ✓ Can you create a demand for your business?
- ✓ Will you follow a marketing plan and stay with it?

In any business, I cannot emphasize enough the importance of having a good business and marketing plan.

In the following chapter the business plan is described fully. There are also many kinds of business plan software available from your local office supply store.

Just remember "**information is power!**" Make it your business to know what business information is available, where to get it and most importantly, how to use it.

CHAPTER 5

WRITING A BUSINESS PLAN

A business plan consists of three main sections, with each section containing specific information about your company's current business and financial position. Here is a brief rundown on each element of a business plan:

1. THE INTRODUCTION:

The introduction consists of about three pages. The first section is intended to give the reader a brief overview of the proposal. The three pages are:

➢ **Title page:** Identifies the company and its principal officers, with name, address, and telephone numbers.

➢ **Table of contents:** Listing the three principal sections and all major subheadings.

➢ **Brief statement:** A brief statement of purpose summarizing the proposal, spelling out how much is involved, and how the funds are to be used. (Ex: 10% marketing, 10% utilities, 50% rent, 20% for loan repayment, 10% office supplies = 100%), how the firm will benefit, and how the funds will be repaid (in the case of a loan).

2. THE DESCRIPTION:

The comments in this section should spell out your company's current business position and its plan for the future. Be certain to address at least five areas of the following in your comments. It should also contain all the steps, which will be taken to get the business started and the direction of where you would like to see the business go in 5 years. It should consist of:

➢ Describing your business in as much detail as possible. Tell what your business is, how you run it, and why you are successful.

➢ Describing your market and your company's market niche. Give some idea of your market's size and potential, and your marketing strategy. Some extra tips to include might be:

1. Identifying the demand for your product/service.

2. Identifying your customers and their location.

3. Explaining how your product and service will be advertised.

4. Discussing how your talent or service will be delivered.

5. Explaining your pricing strategy and your source and amount of initial equity capital.

➢ Developing a monthly operating budget for year 1 and then project out 3 years of quarterly balance sheets and profit and loss statements.

➢ Providing monthly cash flow statements, which tie to the quarterly balance sheets, provided for a 2-year period. Discuss your break-even point and explain your personal balance sheet and method of compensation.

➢ Providing "**what if**" statements to demonstrate alternative approaches to addressing any negative which may develop.

➢ Describing your competition and giving some idea of how you will handle it. Spare no words. If competition is severe, say so. State why your service and product is better than XYZ Billing Service and what extra advantages you are supplying that your competition is not.

➢ Describing your management team, emphasizing the business background and experience of each member of the team. Some personal data, such as age, special interests, and place of residence should be included. Qualifications, past experiences, and future education should be included. Explain the day-to-day operations of the business and discuss future needs to hire and personnel policies and procedures. Mention your lease, insurance, dues, etc. that pertain to your business.

➢ Describing how the new capital will be applied. Spell out what projects the funds will be used for. You should be as specific as possible, which means that you will have to reach some hard decisions before seeking funds.

3. THE FINANCIAL SECTION:

Your "*financial,*" as lenders and other providers of capital commonly label them, should be aimed at providing support for the statements made in the descriptive section.

You will need both historical data and projections for the future. Start off with a Source and Application of Funding statement that shows in detail how the proceeds of the financing will be used (e.g., percentages allocated to equipment, advertising, and product distribution). You can then move on to the more traditional financial statements.

➢ **Historical statements** should go back about 5 years. If you business is cyclical in nature, you should cover a complete cycle, even if it means digging further into the past. The reports should include:

  ✓ balance sheets

  ✓ income statements

  ✓ cash flow statements

➢ **Projections** should also include:

  ✓ Performa balance sheets

  ✓ Income statements

  ✓ Cash-flow statements (summary reports are acceptable in most cases)

Make sure that you include projections for at least the period that the funds will be used and repaid.

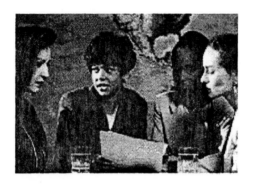

Even though you will usually need a full-blown business plan, running about 12 pages, to ensure proper treatment on most financing expeditions, there are times when a less thorough treatment will do just as well.

You may already have established a close relationship with your bank and merely need to present a documented proposal to the loan committee. Or, you may be attempting to arrange new financing from a private investor who is already familiar with your company's operation. In such cases, a summary financing proposal can usually be substituted for a formal business plan.

A summary financing proposal is a "*mini*" business plan consisting of no more than **six or seven pages.**

The **first page** contains the proposal itself, detailing the amount of cash needed, repayment schedule, collateral, and any other pertinent details.

The **second page** summarizes how the funds will be used and how your firm will benefit. In brief, this section sets forth your arguments on why the proposal will be a good loan or investment.

The second page is followed by a two to three page outline on your company's history, its product and marketing position, its management team, and a summary of its prospects for the future. In short, this is a capsule version of the descriptive section of a formal business plan.

Finally, you should include a condensed balance sheet and income statement, plus a year or two of projections. Cash-flow statements would give you a substantial boost to your argument here.

Once completed, you will now have a clear direction on where you are headed. Some major corporations call this their "**Mission Statement**." Please do not be fooled into thinking this is a waste of time. This will probably be the most *valuable* thing you will ever do.

On my letterhead I have my mission statement which reads:

> *"We are not out to impress our clients,*
> *we are out to amaze them!"*

I use this statement in my marketing materials and emphasize this during my presentations.

FACTS CONCERNING A SMALL BUSINESS:

Taxes - The IRS recommends that you attend a Small Business Tax Workshop. It will provide you with a basic introduction to business taxes.

A WORKSHOP WOULD INCLUDE:

➢ Tax advantages and disadvantages of sole proprietorship.

➢ The basics of preparing your business tax returns.

➢ How to withhold and make deposits of federal taxes.

➢ What records you need and how to keep good records.

➢ The functions of the IRS to include services, tax audits, your appeal rights, and penalties a business may incur.

Discussing your business ideas with your personal accountant will greatly enlighten you to future advantages and future liabilities.

BUSINESS IS LIKE AN AUTOMOBILE.

IT WON'T RUN ITSELF

EXCEPT DOWNHILL!

CHAPTER 6

GETTING STARTED AND NETWORKING

Starting a business can be a trying experience and you will need to get out and meet people and become involved. I know a lot of people who are starting this business and work a full-time job so they won't be able to be as active. However by joining organizations you will get known in the field and you will get free publicity and advertising.

All the organizations I will mention have newsletters, meetings and will possibility write a press release for you. You can join these organizations and they may feature you in their monthly newsletter. What better publicity could you possibility get? And the best part is if you are featured in one of the newsletters, it is free advertising for you.

A lot of these organizations have doctors and dentists who are members. They read newsletters too. By joining, your name is listed in their roster and again, you may be the feature on a newsletter.

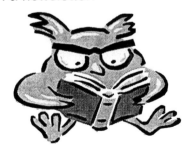

NETWORKING ORGANIZATIONS:

➤ BETTER BUSINESS BUREAU

You will need to be in business for 6 months before you can join but one of the key advantages is that you can use their name on your advertising such as **"Member of the Better Business Bureau."** This presents you as a reputable business. I have had physician practices call the Better Business Bureau to check on my credentials and to see if there were any complaints filed against my company. *My reputation is important and I am proud to be a member of the Better Business Bureau in good standing.*

➤ CHAMBER OF COMMERCE

Have you ever noticed in a physician or dental office a plaque or window sticker saying **"Member of the Chamber of Commerce?"** Many doctors have their membership posted in their office. By joining this organization you will have something in common with the medical profession and again, remember their newsletters. Joining the Chamber of Commerce is another means of networking.

➤ TOASTMASTERS

Are you afraid of the first face to face presentation that you will make? Join Toastmasters and you will get comfortable with public speaking. They also have a newsletter and once more . . . free advertising. They meet early mornings as well as other scheduled times to accommodate the working population.

➤ LOCAL NETWORKING

Check your local papers and see if there are any professional networking luncheons. Some towns have specialized networking luncheons for women groups and minorities. These networking groups are there to help people get ahead in small business. Read your paper carefully and look for groups in your area.

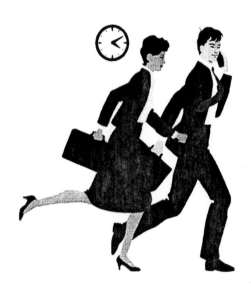

CHAPTER 7

SUPERBILLS AND CLAIM FORMS -

Before we get into marketing and pricing, I would like to make you aware of certain buzzwords. In this business we all use the word *"superbill."* You may ask what is a superbill? A superbill is a printed paper you receive from the physician's office which lists the patient's name and a series of CPT and ICD-9 codes that pertain to that specialty.

The physician will check off the CPT and ICD-9 code that pertain to a particular patient. Some superbills have the patients address, phone number, date of birth and insurance company. An example of a superbill is in Chapter 32. Chapters 26 and 28 will help you to understand the difference between a CPT and ICD-9 code.

When you start billing the physician will give you a copy of their superbill. The superbill is your guide to inputting claims into your practice management software. If you bill for a large practice you will get about 20-30 superbills a day, or possibly more. You will take the superbill information and input the data into your software. Once the information is entered you will not have to reenter the patient data. On repeat visits you will only have to enter the date of service, CPT and ICD-9 code(s). The time involved is less than a minute. The billing software keeps a record of what procedure and diagnosis the physician's office gave you for a particular patient. However, you should keep a copy of the superbill. By law these have to be held for six years.

A HCFA 1500 form is a claim form that is generated from the data you entered in the medical billing software. It is submitted to the insurance company either electronically or on paper. An example HCFA 1500 form is in Chapter 32. If you send a claim on paper you will use the actual HCFA 1500 form and your software will print the form on your printer from the data entered. If you send a claim electronically, your software converts the information you have inputted into the National Standard Format of a HCFA 1500 form and electronically transmits it.

Somewhere in the late 1970's, the American Medical Association (AMA) created a universal claim form that would standardize the information needed by people who are processing the completed claim forms. The HCFA 1500 claim form supplies the information needed to file a claim and includes the patient's data such as date of birth, address, policy identification number, sex, etc. It lists the diagnostic and treatment data along with the provider's identification number and the location of where the services were provided (hospital, nursing home, physician office, etc.). There is a list of place of service codes in your software.

An *Explanation of Benefits (EOB)* is a detailed summary of the direct payment to the health care provider from the insurance company. The EOB will list the patient's name, procedure, allowable fee and the fee submitted from the provider's office. It will also list denials or deductibles as the reason for denial or duplication of a particular claim. An example EOB is in Chapter 32.

As you read the next chapter you will get a brief summary of books available that will further help you to understand the medical claims process.

CHAPTER 8

REFERENCE BOOKS

Before we begin the reference section, let's understand why reference books give us essential information. When physicians see patients, they report and submit a HCFA 1500 claim form, either on paper or electronically, to the insurance company. The claim form will contain all the necessary information as well as the reason the patient was seen (using a CPT code) and why (using an ICD-9 code).

A procedure (commonly called CPT codes) is a listing of description terms and identifying codes for reporting medical services and procedures performed by a physician. It could be for a common cold. If that were the case, they would code the procedure as an Evaluation & Management. A patient could be seen for the removal of a wart, which would then become a procedure that would be coded as a Surgical Procedure. And the list goes on and on.

Once a procedure is determined, a diagnosis (called ICD 9-CM codes) must be determined which will tell the insurance company the reason for the procedure, service, or supply. An example of a diagnosis is whooping cough, immunity deficiency, hemorrhaging, etc.

PROCEDURES ARE GROUPED IN SIX MAJOR SECTIONS:

- ➢ Medicine
- ➢ Evaluation & Management (E/M)
- ➢ Anesthesiology
- ➢ Pathology & Laboratory
- ➢ Surgery
- ➢ Radiology

After the doctor codes the procedure from one of the six sections above he needs to indicate a diagnosis code. Diagnosis codes are broken into subsections according to body part, service, or diagnosis (ex: mouth, amputation or septal defect). A diagnosis is used for indexing the specific reason, such as the classification of the disease (ex: acute conjunctivas, unspecified osteomyelitis, or urinary tract infection). The diagnosis code will tell the insurance company what the reason for the visit was.

An example would be the physician sees a patient in his office and uses the Evaluation and Management **procedure code** of 99212 which is for an office visit 20 minutes in length. He discovers the patient has a urinary tract infection therefore his **diagnosis code** would be 599.9. This information is transferred to the insurance company.

St. Anthony's, Medical Arts Press and PMIC are three excellent companies to purchase **ICD-9** and **CPT** books from. These books are also essential to perform proper medical billing. When you purchase the books, read carefully and thoroughly the Preface of the books and any other pertinent information the book may have. Many changes occur each year and this information will be highlighted in the book. The books also explain what certain symbols mean and the meaning of color codes.

I have purchased books from Medical Arts Press (800-826-6706), PMIC (1-800-MED-SHOP) and MediCode (801-536-1000). All the companies are excellent in their customer service department. There are other companies out there. You may want to shop around to various book companies for the best prices.

Medical Arts Press will set up an account and bill you later. They are located in Minneapolis, Minnesota. PMIC wants a Visa or Master Card before sending you the books.

The two books that I feel are absolutely necessary are the ICD 9-CM and CPT code books. Some other books you may want to consider are "*Understanding Medical Insurance*" by Joanne C. Rowell which can be purchased from PMIC or Medical Arts Press and "*Code It Right*" which can be purchased from MediCode (801-536-1000).

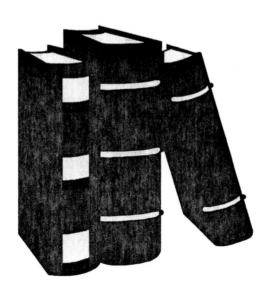

I have listed the following books that I feel will be a great guide to help you in successfully submitting claims.

➢ **ICD 9-CM** (Listing of all diagnostic codes)

> You will need an **ICD 9-CM**, Volume 1 and 2. An **ICD 9-CM** is the coding book used by physicians. All physicians are required by law to submit diagnosis codes for reimbursement.
>
> **ICD** stands for **International Classification of Diseases.** It is also known as the coding system physicians must use. The book I use is the St. Anthony's book. It is expensive, but they supply you with updates for a full year. Coding books need to be <u>kept current</u> and accurate. There are changes throughout the year that you must be aware of and you will need to update regularly.

➢ **CPT** (Listing of all procedure codes)

> **CPT** stands for **Current Procedural Terminology**. It is a listing of descriptive terms and identifying codes for reporting medical services and procedures performed by physicians.
>
> The purpose of the terminology is to provide a uniform language that will describe medical, surgical, and diagnostic services accurately.
>
> The codes serve a wide variety of important functions. It is also useful for administrative management purposes such as claims processing.

➤ **CDT-2** (A code book designed specifically for dental billing)

➤ **HCPCS** (More specific means of coding to include modifiers)

> HCPC is an acronym for **Health Care Financing Administration Common Procedure Coding System.** The pronunciation for HCPCS is "hick-picks."
>
> This system is a uniform method for healthcare providers and medical suppliers to report professional services, procedures, and supplies. This book not only enables the operational needs of Medicare/Medicaid, it coordinates government programs by uniform application of HCFA **(Health Care Financing Administration)** policies, and allows providers and suppliers to communicate their services in a consistent manner. This book is a necessary part of your library.

Additional books worth having are:

➤ *Insurance Directory*

> Although you can survive without this book, the Insurance Directory designed by Medicode, provides the most complete, accurate, and up-to-date demographic information on insurance payers across the country. You will find examples of forms for use in your office. The book provides information regarding how insurers pay claims as well as how you should submit and monitor those claims.

➤ **Reimbursement Manual for the Medical Office**

Guides you through each step of the reimbursement process. Covers terminology, CPT, HCPCS and ICD 9-CM, billing processes, forms, fee setting, superbill design, plus dealing with insurance carriers and managed care organizations (HMOs/PPOs).

➤ **Medicare Rules & Regulations**

Contains material from the official Medicare Carriers Manual.

➤ **Medical Marketing Handbook**

Designed to help simplify the concepts and strategies of medical marketing. This book helps develop a comprehensive marketing plan for medical management.

➤ **Medical Acronyms, Eponyms & Abbreviations**

This guide helps you translate those tricky acronyms and abbreviations. Covers all medical specialties plus nursing, administration, quality assurance, dietetics, pharmacy and lab.

➤ **Law, Liability, and Ethics for Medical Office Personnel**

If you don't understand all the laws that impact a practice, this book clearly depicts the statutes and regulations that affect today's medical practices.

There are many more books available than those that I mentioned. Call PMIC. MediCode and Medical Arts Press. Ask them to send you their catalog free of charge and to put you on their mailing list for specials.

HCFA forms can be purchased from almost any company. I purchase my forms from Moore at 708-913-3200. At the time they were the least expensive, although that too changes daily. I believe PMIC, and Medical Arts Press may carry them as well as MediSoft.

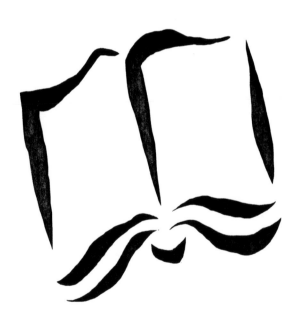

CHAPTER 9

WHAT DOCTORS WANT TO HEAR

It has been said that many doctors prefer to keep to the practice of medicine and allow office staff or accountants to handle the financial part of their business. Harvard University is contemplating a mandatory course where all doctors will have to start taking some business management courses. Physicians have their expertise in their field of study to be the very best they can; however, the bottom line is "they need more business/financial orientation," which you as a billing center may be able to provide.

Doctors want to **hear how you can save them money** and that you have the ability to file their claims quickly and accurately so they can get their money promptly. By filing electronically you can cut the accounts receivable turnaround time from 28 or more to 7-21 days. They want to hear that you can file their claims with a 97% accuracy rate.

One thing physicians do not know is that most office managers may give up on claims after they are rejected several times. This is a frustrating process because the time involved in reprocessing claims can be tedious and prevents the office staff from submitting current claims or keeping abreast of general office duties. Don't ever criticize their office manager for this. Physicians do not want you coming in and telling them their office management team are not sufficient.

Unfortunately the physician never finds out about those lost claims. In this business we call those claims the *"Mercedes or Porsche"* drawer. It would be a shame to count the thousands of dollars that are disregarded because office personnel either don't want to or are too busy to look for old EOB's or surgical reports to attach and resubmit. Another reason claims go into the Mercedes or Porsche drawer is due to changes in office personnel.

Whatever the reason, if you can discretely convince the physician that this is happening in his practice, you may have a new client. I told one physician about the Mercedes drawer and she asked me what a Mercedes drawer was. After I explained, she called me back that night and said she never thought about a Mercedes drawer but realized that was happening.

The bottom line is, don't put the office manger/staff down because the physician may think the staff is the best thing that ever happened to their practice. Convince the physician that their office management is best suited to take care of their patients and their needs, and should not be distracted by the mundane billing and insurance process.

If possible, try and be up on the latest news with Medicare and other health insurance companies. I always advise my trainees before meeting with a physician that they should spend time on the internet and learn as much about the specialty as possible. If you made it this far to meet with the physician – be confident and as knowledgeable as possible. You may also want to network with your fellow peers before the meeting. If possible, find out what procedures Medicare won't pay for.

When the physician gives you their superbill, you will be able to look at it and tell them which services are not covered or which procedures are no longer accepted.

A TRUE STORY -

I had a client in California. When I met with him and we studied his physician's superbill, the first thing I recognized was a surgical code that was deleted two years prior. This proved to be a valuable asset to my client. He was then able to explain to the physician why the claim forms were constantly being denied.

This proves another example of how the office staff was not able to keep current with the latest changes.

When reviewing a superbill you may notice a procedure that is coded incorrectly. The physician may ask you to code the patient differently. In order to do this, the physician must have documented notes in the patient chart to justify the change in codes. You, as a medical specialist are not certified to code. You can only recommend that a code needs to be changed. Your job is not to code but to file claims; however you may recommend how a physician can optimize proper coding on his superbill. Again, this is an example of the importance of being familiar with the physician's specialty. This will demonstrate your knowledge and expertise in the field.

Another area you should gain knowledge in is the number of authorized visits for various procedures that are allowed by insurance carriers. You can call your Medicare/Medicaid office in your state to gain information about the limitation on the number of visits for various procedures.

If the physician asks you a question that you cannot answer, be honest. Tell the physician you do not have the answer, but will get back to him with the correct information as soon as possible.

Physicians want to hear that you can help make their practice function more efficiently by outsourcing their medical billing and allowing their staff to concentrate on the needs of their patients. The physician wants to be assured that you are reliable and capable and can maximize their cash flow by timely submission of their insurance claims. Convince the physician that the success of your business is dependent on the success of their practice.

The bottom line . . . you need to emphasize that collecting their insurance payments promptly and efficiently will be a reflection on your company, and therefore you will work hard for them.

Additionally, you want the physician to know:

➢ You can improve cash flow, in most cases by 97%.

➢ You are consistent - an average physician's employee turns over every 2.6 years. That means the physician would have to hire and train new staff that will cost time and money.

➢ Using a billing service is cost effective - the average practice that files by paper spends between $6 - $12 a claim, you can do it electronically for $3.00 or less per claim.

➢ By using a billing service the physician does not have to be concerned with employee vacations, sick days, or holidays. You are there and are reliable.

➢ Emphasize, you are an extension of the physician's office - just a phone call away.

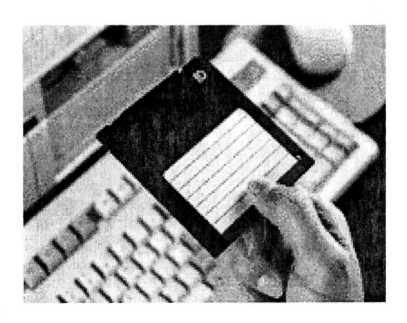

CHAPTER 10

PRICING YOUR SERVICES

Correctly pricing your services in your geographic area is very important. Therefore I suggest you try and obtain your competitor's fees and also be aware that medical specialists in different parts of the country charge different rates. Also be aware that pricing may differ for various physicians specialties.

Fees are also dependent on whether you want to have a Full Service Billing Center or submitting claims only.

Full-Service Billing Centers Include:

➢ Submitting claims electronically and on paper when necessary.

➢ Patient ledgers - shows patient activity such as charges, payments, and account adjustments. An account adjustment could be Capitation because of an HMO or PPO.

Remember Capitation is an agreement between the physician and HMO/ PPO that refers to a set amount of money that the doctor and the insurance company agree upon. An example would be an HMO/PPO will only pay an agreed upon fee to the physician for service rendered for each individual patient, whether that patient is seen by the physician or not.

The physician will still receive the agreed upon fee even if the patient is seen numerous times during the year. In comparison to a physician who is not part of a HMO/PPO, this could result in a loss for the HMO/PPO physician. By law the difference between what the physician is charging, and what an HMO/PPO pays, cannot be collected from the patient.

➢ Patient statements - is what the billing service will send to the patient when you bill them for balances that are usually not covered by the insurance company.

➢ Management reports - are reports you give to the doctors and can include any one or all of the following:

    ✓ Insurance analysis report
    ✓ Capitation reports
    ✓ An analysis of the practice that gives the doctor information on procedures, payments received and accounts.
    ✓ An outstanding balance sheet on what is owed and what has been billed for a particular month or year.
    ✓ Visit report - showing the doctor the number of visits allowed and the number of visits used for insurance purposes.

The fee for full-service billing varies from 5-12% of what is collected from the insurance companies. You can call around to different billing centers in your area and find out what the going rate for your area is.

Prospective medical billing specialists ask me how I feel about charging a set-up fee. A lot is dependent on how the meeting is going and what the competition is. I don't generally charge a set-up fee for a small practice however, if the practice were large I would surely charge a set-up fee. Set-up fees vary from $100 - $500 or more.

A TRUE STORY

Someone I know investigated the billing centers in their area by saying they were an accountant for a physician and was checking on billing centers to see if it were feasible for their client. The billing centers, thinking they were getting a client, were happy to give that individual whatever information they needed. The main objective here is to find out their fee and ask them to mail you an information packet. This will give you a comparison as to what your competition is.

CLAIMS ONLY

A claim only is submitting "only claims" and is different from full service billing. The average fee for a per-claim submission is anywhere from $1.50 per claim to $15.00 a claim, depending on specialty. Again, if you call your competitor (another billing center) and find out their rate you will have a guideline to go by. This will greatly aid you in keeping your services in the competitive market. Again, area and location will depend on pricing your services. Billing in the Northeast could be substantially different from that of the Southeast. Have knowledge of your competitor's fees.

In pricing your services, it is unlikely you would charge $4.00 per claim if the claim only takes you a minute to input. A more reasonable fee would be $1.50 per claim per minute which equates to over $50 an hour. This is explained further in this chapter. Again, you need to remain competitive in your geographical area.

When a claim is submitted and the claim is rejected because of an office error you can charge a physician an additional fee to resubmit the claim; however, if the mistake is yours and not the physicians, **I don't recommend charging the additional fee.**

A lot may depend on your clearinghouse as well. Some clearinghouses charge an additional submission fee to resubmit a claim, while other clearinghouses reject a claim immediately and the resubmission is free.

The bottom line is your fee will be determined by what kind of specialty you are billing for and how many claims you can input in an hour. If you are billing for a physician who has a repeat business and the claims never really change much and you are entering a claim a minute, your fee would be much lower. In that case you would charge at the low end of the scale.

When you analyze the kind of business you would like to have (Full-Service vs. Claims only) you need to consider the extra expenses of using the phone, calling insurance companies, spending money on postage, letterhead, envelopes, etc. Additionally, you need to consider your workload. You need to discuss with the physician whether or not you will be using his stationary and envelopes or supplying them yourself. That will also help you in determining your fee schedule. Once you can project your expenses you will then have an educated decision on what your charges should be.

Generally speaking, most billing centers price out their services to approximately $50.00 an hour for work provided, whether it is full billing or per claim submission. Again, your hourly fee is based on geographic location and competitors fees.

FREE TRIAL

Free trials are another marketing tool that many billing centers use. I don't recommend a free trial. What I do recommend is a reduced rate for 3 months to see how the working relationship is surviving and it also gives you an excellent opportunity to track your time and expenses. This will enable you to see if your fee is too high or too low. During the presentation I tell the physician that at the end of the three months period we will renegotiate the fee if necessary. This is also a good time to talk about changes such as adding or deleting services and to ensure that the physician is happy with the services they are receiving.

One thing prospective entrepreneurs ask me is *"How much money can I make?"* There are many factors involved to determine how much money can be made. Some of those factors are:

- ✓ The type of specialty you are billing for
- ✓ The amount of claims the provider is submitting
- ✓ The gross amount of money the physician brings in
- ✓ The amount of accounts you have
- ✓ The amount of time you are investing per account

An example would be XYZ Billing Center is billing for a physician that brings in over $300,000 a year. You are billing for a practice that brings in $100,000 a year. You and XYZ Billing Center are charging 7% and are both investing equal time. It is easy to calculate that the difference in the 300,000 vs. the 100,000 @ 7% is significant.

The bottom line on billing is that you wouldn't charge a doctor $3.00 a claim if that claim takes you less than a minute to input. There are variations with every practice and with all data entry.

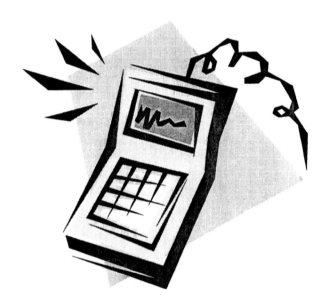

A quick crash course in pricing your services:

Dr. Guido filed 200 claims a month with the average claim being $100. (Total monthly income would be $20,000 in submitted insurance claims). It takes you approximately 2 minutes to enter a claim. How much would you charge?

	333.50
Flat Fee	_____
	1.67
Per Claim	_____
	1.7%
%	_____

First off let's assume you want to make $50 an hour.

To Figure Your Flat Fee -
You would take the 200 claims and multiply that by 2 minutes and come up with 400 minutes or 6.67 hours. At $50 an hour you would multiply 6.67 by $50 and your time would be worth $333.50 a month to file 200 claims.

To Figure Your Per Claim -
You divide the $333.50 by 200 claims and you would get $1.67 a claim.

To Figure Your Percentage -
Divide $20,000 by $333.50 and you come up with .016% which when rounded off, comes to 1.7% which equals $340 monthly.

You have now calculated your flat and per claim fee as well as your percentage. You will then need to adjust the fee higher to cover your expenses.

Dr. Dion billed out $100,000 a month and saw approximately 500 patients per month (average bill $200.). It takes you about 4 minutes to file the claim. What would you charge?

Flat fee

$1666.50

_____

Per Claim

$ 3.33

_____

%

1.66%

_____

To Figure Your Flat Fee –

➢ You take 500 claims x 4 minutes to come up with 2,000 minutes or 33.33 hours.
➢ At $50 an hour you multiply $50. x 33.33 hours = $1,666.50 as a flat fee.

To Figure Your Per Claim

➢ You divide $1666.50 by 500 claims to come up with $3.33 a claim.

To Figure Your %

➢ You take $100,000 divided by $1666.50 and get 1.66

You are now able to give the physician 3 options of billing. Presenting the three options allows the physician the opportunity of what outsourcing will be costing as compared to having a full or part time biller in the physician office.

Billing on a percentage is to the physicians advantage because you will work harder knowing that every dollar that comes in is part of your percentage. I myself would much rather work on a percentage. I find myself eager to post payments knowing that I am getting a percent of what is posted.

Again when pricing your services, be sure to take into consideration the following expenses and incorporate them in your fee.

✓ Initial set-up expenses

✓ Office overhead/your overhead

✓ Advertising

✓ How often you pick up information

✓ How far you will be traveling

✓ Office supplies

✓ Phone charges

✓ Meetings

~ THE BOTTOM LINE ~

WHAT IS YOUR TIME WORTH?

YOU CAN ALWAYS START HIGH AND COME DOWN –

YOU CAN'T START LOW AND COME UP!

CHAPTER 11

MARKETING STRATEGIES

YOUR KEY TO MARKETING YOUR SERVICES

Marketing is the most important part of your business. Without a proper marketing plan and continuous marketing strategies your business will eventually decay. You need to be prepared to follow your marketing plan and **budget marketing expenses faithfully.**

Let's assume you were planning a trip across the country. The first thing you would do is purchase a map of the states you plan on visiting, then you would mark your destination. Marketing a business is very similar. You need to know how you will get from point A to point B. You don't need too many details, just an easy plan on how you are getting there. The same thing goes for your business . . . you need to think of your goals, your finances and your projected time frame and determine what it will take to get there. You need to plan a budget of expenses, and you need to follow that plan.

A GOOD MARKETING PLAN

SHOULD

NOT BE FLEXIBLE.

Different types of marketing are radio, newspaper, magazines, television, direct mail, cold-calling, yellow pages, brochures, telephone marketing, trade shows, public relations, press release, and most importantly, word of mouth and referrals.

DIRECT MAIL

The most common type, although not the most effective, is direct mail since most people hate the "*cold-call approach*." You can obtain a book of computerized information that will include doctors by states and their individual specialty from your local library. CAY Medical Management offers a listing of 500 physicians in your area presently not filing claims electronically for $175. You can reach them at 800-221-0488. Your local Medicare office also has a listing free of charge. These lists are free however they take approximately six weeks or more to obtain and many people find the hassle of getting to the right person to request the list not worth their time.

You need to market these physicians a minimum of three times to get your name out. I suggest in my marketing class that if you were to target 300 physicians in a three-month period, you would be marketing to 25 physicians a week. You would then consistently send out the same 25 mailings for twelve consecutive weeks until all the 300 physicians received the same direct mail marketing material.

After the twelve weeks design another marketing material and re-market those same 300 physicians which would take another twelve weeks. After the 2nd twelve-week period re-market once again with a third type of mailing.

By doing this, your name is getting out. Your marketing may be filed away for future use or at one point the office may decide they would like to outsource. Hopefully since you had sent marketing material three times to them they will remember your name and call you. By following this scenario you not only are being consistent but you are staying within a budget. If your budget allows you can double the number.

Decide your strategy, draw your road map on how you would like to get there, and follow it through faithfully while staying within budget. Don't quit after one or two months. Be persistent! If you decide you want to take another route in marketing, finish out your original plan first before you decide to switch direction. You need to be consistent in your marketing strategies.

COLD CALLING

Cold calling is the most effective means of marketing. If you are cold calling remember the old rule is for every 20 no's you will get one yes. In this business it may be for every 50 no's, you will get a yes.

Don't get discouraged. You are selling a service! Eventually you will find a person who is in need of that service. Take packets with you the day you cold-call and if you get a foot in the door *leave a packet.* Otherwise, take brochures with you and leave them with the receptionist. If you can get the name of the office manager, leave the brochure and call her back in a few days. Make sure on the day you cold-call you look your best. It is a proven fact that you need to dress for success.

Cold calling is the most effective way to getting an appointment and without a doubt, it is the *least expensive* way of marketing. Some people consider cold calling the most difficult of marketing strategies. Everyone has different feelings about it. My friend Sally in Texas loves to cold call while I would be terrified. If you know a sales person who has been trained to do this get some tips. You may even consider taking a friend with you. Just be comfortable in your decision.

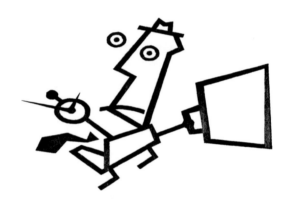

THE FIVE STEPS TO COLD CALLING ARE:

- Get the attention of the person

- Identify yourself and your company

- The reason for the call

- A qualifying or questioning statement

- Setting the appointment

A physician's office that requests more data is possibly your first step in obtaining a client. Try offering the physician/office manager your brochure and an opportunity to come back for a "*free consultation.*" This offer may get you an appointment. At the appointment, which is the actual meeting, you are on a personal basis and it is the time to then sell yourself and your service.

There are also some words that we refer to as "***buzz***" words on the following pages. Use them in your vocabulary and brochures.

The following words will carry a lot of weight. Use them often. They are:

Introducing	*Free*	*New*
Save	*Money*	*Discover*
Results	*Easy*	*Proven*
Guaranteed	*Benefits*	*Alternative*
Trustworthy	*Comfortable*	*Proud*
Safe	*Security*	*Winnings*
Value	*Announcing*	*Advice*
Why	*Your*	*People*

Words which could be intimidating, and I suggest not to use are:

Buy	*Obligation*	*Failure*
Bad	*Sell*	*Loss*
Difficult	*Wrong*	*Decision*
Deal	*Liability*	*Hard*
Contract	*Fail*	*Cost*

Chapter 12

Newspapers

Following the Help Wanted Ads

You can either place an ad about your service in the local newspaper or you can follow the classifieds. Every time you see an advertisement for a medical billing specialist, send them your brochure and a cover letter.

There have been many successful medical billing centers that were able to get started by following the Sunday classifieds.

Analyze the example on the next page. You may want to change it. Consider any modifications that you feel may be appropriate for your business.

EXAMPLE OF A BUSINESS COVER LETTER -

XYZ Billing Center
3 Billing Center Drive
Anytown, USA 03039

800-212-2345

June 11, 1999

Dr. Richard Casey
3 Physicians Lane
Physician City, New York 83839

Dear Dr. Casey:

I would like to introduce myself and my billing service. I am an independent billing service that files insurance claims electronically. My experience includes years of medical billing and claims processing, as well as hospital administration. I attend conferences to remain aware of continuous changes in the healthcare industry.

When you read through the enclosed material, you will understand that it is far more advantageous for you to utilize our services to file your Medicaid/Medicare and commercial claims, than to have your staff perform in house medical billing.

If you were paying an employee $8 an hour based on a 20 hour week, you have already spent $160.00 in salary for a week, or $8,320 a year. In addition you are also paying for benefits such as vacation, sick days, and holidays. Let your office staff concentrate on extraordinary patient care.

XYZ Billing Service will submit your claims efficiently, provide your office with reports and not call in sick, take vacation days, and spend your money making personal calls. Your success is our number one priority.

I would welcome the opportunity to sit and meet with you and present you with a cost comparison. I will also show you how we can submit your claims fast and in the most expedient way. Feel free to contact me at your convenience.

Sincerely,

Sally Dodge

ANOTHER EXAMPLE OF A COVER LETTER YOU MAY CONSIDER SENDING IN RESPONSE TO THE "HELP WANTED ADS."

XYZ Billing Center
3 Billing Center Drive
Anytown, USA 03039

800-212-2345

June 11, 1999

Dr. Richard Casey
3 Physicians Lane
Physician City, New York 83839

Dear Dr. Casey:

Statistics show that even if your staff is consistent in resubmitting insurance claims, the time it takes you to receive insurance payments may take months.   This means that your cash flow is seeping away. The federally enacted Omnibus Reconciliation Act requires you to file your patients' Medicare/Medicaid forms.   Filing claims manually result in account errors. When claims are filed electronically they have a 97% accuracy rate. What that means to you is that the claims are made payable before they are submitted. It also means you will see a faster return on your money. XYZ can significantly reduce the time it takes for you to be paid, from months to days, often only two weeks.

XYZ Billing Service has the capability to electronically file claims for private insurance carriers, as well as

Medicare/Medicaid. Although you may be filing Medicare claims on a computer and then printing the claims out on a HCFA form to mail, this is not considered electronic filing, it is manual paper submission. Electronic claims are processed ahead of paper claims!

We're experienced, confident and dedicated to providing your practice with electronic claims processing system. Your staff may be spending a lot of time and money rectifying the insurance claims nightmare. If that is the case, XYZ Billing Service is your solution. The time to act is now!

Should you have any questions, please contact my office so that I may provide more information on our state of the art claims processing system.

Sincerely,

Sally Dodge
President
XYZ Billing Service

CHAPTER 13

DIRECT MARKETING:

PRESS RELEASES -
HOSPITALS -
ADVERTISING -
YELLOW PAGES -

PRESS RELEASES

Have you ever wondered about your daily newspaper and the "Who's Who in Business" section? Look for it. See what they say. Try writing a press release about your business and send it to the newspapers in your area/state.

An example might start with:

"Mrs. Sally Dodge of XYZ Billing Service has opened a Medical Billing service in the area".

Then you proceed to tell something about yourself that would be an asset.

If you are already in business write a press release anyway.

"Mrs. Sally Dodge is expanding her services to include electronic dental submission!"

I'm sure when you look at the press releases in your newspapers you can write an essay on yourself. If you have no prior experience in the field, go on to say:

Sally Dodge is the parent of three and a little league coach. She recently attended training at the Academy of Medical Billing and is a member of the Better Business Bureau.

I think by now you understand what I am saying. The best part is that a press release is free advertising. What better way is there to get the word out?

HOSPITALS

Call or write the hospitals in your area, ask them if you can set up a table to be available for physicians and/or office managers to discuss the advantages of electronic medical claims submission. Some hospitals will allow you to use the cafeteria. Once you have made all your arrangements and established a place in the hospital send out flyers to area physicians telling them the specifics of where you are and date and time. You might even want to publish this information in a press release.

If you have the means available, be ready to give a "free cost analysis."

If you know someone that works in a hospital you might try asking them to leave your brochure or flyer in the physician's lounge. Usually physicians will be in the lounge between surgery and going over paperwork with a cup of coffee. If your brochure is appealing, they will pick it up.

If you cannot get a hospital to give you space for a table you may consider doing this in a hotel.

ADVERTISING

Call your local American Medical Association (AMA). Inquire about advertising in their monthly newsletter. The advertising fee will vary depending on what kind of ad you place. When I started out I was very successful with my advertising ad. I chose a block ad.

The advertisement can be as simple as –

POOR CASH FLOW

Is this disease killing your practice?

Signs: **High Receivables, Low Income**

Symptoms: **Aging over 45 days. Chronic claim denials**

TREATMENT: **XYZ Billing Service**

XYZ takes the claims you've given up on and get the money you've already earned – FAST

Call 800-XYZ-SALLY

With a little imagination you can write a great ad, but remember to "keep it simple." Give them enough information to stir their curiosity to call you.

My marketing in the AMA Newsletter was very successful. The physicians will call you and not be on the defensive. You are providing a service they are interested in.

A word of caution – be prepared with a script near the telephone to answer direct questions when they do call.. You will not know when the call comes in so be prepared.

A TRUE STORY –

When I received my first call from a physician responding to my AMA newsletter ad I was flustered, nervous and unprepared for the call. I repeated myself, gave an unrealistic percentage quote without gathering information and lost the proposed client. I learned the hard way and finally prepared a script to keep nearby.

YELLOW PAGES

List your business telephone as a business with your local telephone company. The fee is slightly higher but you are then entitled to a free listing in the yellow pages in your local phone book. Not only is the free listing important but you would also be listed in the information directory. If a prospective client misplaces your telephone number, the probability is they would remember your business name and obtain your number from the information directory.

CHAPTER 14

DIRECT MAIL
POSTCARDS –
BROCHURES –
LETTERS –

If cold calling is not for you another successful way of marketing is through direct mail. This may be easier however it is more expensive. **Remember your marketing budget.**

You can mail postcards, brochures and letters. Marketing statistics with the postcard approach are relatively good. When you mail a questionnaire postcard, the physician's office may take several minutes and fill out the questionnaire and mail it back to you. This is discussed further in the chapter.

The brochure/letter approach is also a good method. The brochure will have statistics and information about your service. The letter approach will explain your services. If the physician is in need or having problems with his billing, then he may be very anxious to outsource his billing.

If your not receiving much response from your direct mailings don't get discouraged. In 2-3 months send back another type of marketing to the same practices. If you decide to use the phone book, I suggest you don't send individual mailings to each physician in a group practice. You are wasting your <u>money</u> because one letter to the practice/office manager should be sufficient.

I have seen great results marketing with a flyer on a paper with a colored border around the edge. You can find that kind of paper in Staples or from 1-800-A-PAPERS. Areas that you normally would bring attention with bold font would be highlighted in bold color to match the same color as the bordered paper. A trainee of mine did her marketing that way and contracted with four physicians in a month. Two of the physicians told her they were quite impressed with her marketing because it stood apart from her competitors.

Other marketing ideas would be limiting your marketing to small practices or specialties (chiropractors, podiatry, psychologist, psychiatrist, and ambulance companies). Whatever your ideas you have to test the market in your area. You may want to call your phone company and get a phone book for every town/city in your state. Most of the phone companies will supply it free of charge. This will give you more names of providers to market throughout your state.

Send 25-100 postcards, letters or brochures a week, depending on your budget and your allowable time. Although many people do not follow-up on their mailings, follow-up is the key to marketing. If you are sending out a survey letter or postcard with a return, statistics show that the return is less than 2%. On my mailings I experienced a higher return rate of 4-8%.

I cannot reiterate enough . . . this business will take time, perseverance and patience. If your return is less than 2%, don't become defeated. Be aware that many mailings do not go directly to the physician. The office staff could discard your mailings if they feel it is a threat. Joseph Kennedy once said:

"You can't learn to win until you learn to lose"

Remember for every 20 no's you will finally get a yes.

POSTCARD MAILING

Pages 90 and 91 is an example of the postcard approach.

The post-card is perforated for easy tearing. Hopefully the physician's office will read the postcard and mail back the return questionnaire survey quickly.

The expense involved in sending postcards is that you need to pre-stamp the return card for their convenience. It can get extremely costly, so limit yourself to 25-100 a week (depending on your budget and again, your marketing plan). Many people have had great success in sending out the postcard survey questionnaire.

Study the postcard carefully. Did you notice there isn't anything on the postcard indicating which physicians office is filling out the questionnaire survey card and mailing it back to you? The reason is simple. The physician office is more likely to fill out the postcard and answer the questionnaire survey because they may not feel that they are responding to a billing center and therefore it poses no threat.

I recommend that you develop a method to code each postcard questionnaire survey card with each practice you send it to. I coded each postcard with a number in small print in the corner of the return postcard. I then had a notebook where I recorded the code applying it to a physician name. An example of this is - Dr. Smith will be #1 in the book and #1 on the postcard, Dr. Jim will be #2 in the book and #2 on the postcard and so on. The coding of the postcards is important so that you can determine who the replying physician is.

On the other hand, you may want to have your name, address and phone number on the card. It is a matter of personal preference. The decision between having your name on the card or not is your choice.

TRUE STORY –

My first client was pricing various billing agencies and he responded to my postcard approach. I didn't have my telephone number on the card therefore he returned it asking me to call him. To this day I still have my first client and now put my telephone number on the post card.

Another tip on postcard mailings is to have the cards professionally printed which will cost about $80 per 1,000. A lot of feedback that I have received from my trainees is that they have experienced success based on the professionally designed postcard. Types of paper such as light blue or pink linen with your logo may possibly make a great difference in your marketing success.

Carefully study the postcard on page 90 and 91. You may need to cut and paste to determine what your final product will look like. Fold it several times, make sure the wording is correct and not upside down. Did you notice there is still one side that has no wording? Be creative and add some inspiring message or logo. You may even want to consider a "fact" about your billing service or your mission statement. But remember to get it right.

TRUE STORY –

My first attempt at a postcard was a disaster. I had it printed all wrong and it was my own fault for not laying it out properly. I knew what I wanted and thought the printer knew what I wanted, only to find out later that the postcards were printed wrong. My only recourse was to separate every card.

Unfortunately, sometimes we assume that the printer understands exactly what we are thinking and that may not be the case. If your final product does not look or fold correctly it is probably your mistake. You wasted your own money.

Sample postcard Side A

Doctors Address
Goes Here

place
your
stamp
here

Your full
billing address
goes here

Fold with easy perforation goes here

We would greatly appreciate you taking the time to answer and return this stamped postcard of survey questions concerning medical insurance claims.

	YES	NO
Do you process medical insurance forms for your patients?	☐	☐
Do you use computerized means to process and send Medical insurance claims to carriers (Medicare, BCBC, and Private carriers)?	☐	☐
Do you contract with someone to process your medical insurance?	☐	☐
Are your accounts receivable at 30 days?	☐	☐
Would you like to receive information on available claims processing services?	☐	☐

THANK YOU FOR YOUR TIME.
Questions please call 800-123-4567

XYZ BILLING SERVICE
Electronic Claims & Practice Management
800-123-4567

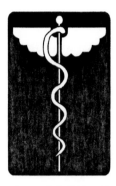

THE
PRESCRIPTION
TO MANAGING
HEALTH CARE
PRACTICES
OF THE 90'S

Print Name
_____

Address
_____

City   State   Zip

XYZ BILLING SERVICE
143 NORTH BILLING CIRCLE
ANYTOWN, USA 03030-0909

BROCHURE/LETTER APPROACH

There are many other ways of getting your foot in the physician's office. I know quite a few people who have sent out brochures with a cover letter and were quite successful. You can create your own brochure with minimum skill using a computer. There are all sorts of helpful aids including an inexpensive Color Bubble Jet Printer for colorful marketing.

I created my brochures with Microsoft Publisher. I used many of the products and templates that Paper Direct offered. Paper Direct has a large array of paper products to aid you in your advertising. Call Paper Direct at 1-800-A-PAPERS and get on their mailing list. They offer a packet of samples of their different stationary. I found that Paper Directs unique design printed papers are the easiest and the least expensive way to add the impact of color to your brochures and stationary.

When you print your own brochures you have the flexibility to print as few or as many as needed. You can save money by making your own brochures that can look just as professional as if you were to have a printer do them. You need to adjust and modify a brochure fully until you feel comfortable with sending it out. You may decide to use one of the sample letters in this booklet to send with your brochure. Try sending a brochure with or without the letter. You need to test your market.

Remember you will have to mail again to these doctors in three months.

Sending a brochure with a survey letter is another way to market. Don't make your marketing materials in a hurry. Spend time on them, look at them, examine for errors, and lastly, sleep on it. The next day carefully review what you have created and see if you can improve it. Make sure your letter and brochure are in superb condition. Don't forget, as with cold calling this brochure may lead you to an appointment.

I have given you an example of my brochure on the next page. I'm sure you have a lot of good ideas you'll want to incorporate into your brochure. Get other people's brochures, study them, compare, change and add.

Once you have your brochure the way you want it, give it to your family and friends. Ask for constructive criticism. You may change your brochure many times before the finished product is completed but I'm sure it will look great.

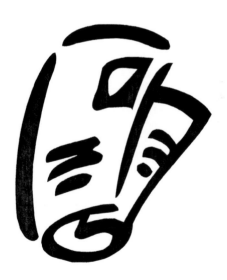

Someday
ALL
HealthCare claims will be
processed electronically.
It will save you time and
money.

Shouldn't you start
saving that
time and money
TODAY?

The money you save is
yours,
not the
insurance company's.

Invest your savings in
your future!

Our mission is not

to satisfy our clients . . . .

but to amaze them!

Who Is CAY Medical Management?

Claudia Yalden, president and owner of CAY Medical Management, Inc. realized the need for Electronic Data Interchange (EDI). She left her position at Children's Hospital in Boston, Massachusetts where she managed the Child Development Unit for Dr. T. Berry Brazelton, author of the best selling book *"Touchpoints"* and Emmy Award winner of his own daytime series *"What Every Baby Knows."*

Claudia formed her own company in 1992 to pursue her dream of owning and operating a medical billing center. She is the author of the newly published book *"Medical Billing . . . The Bottom Line"* and founder of *The Academy of Medical Billing.* Her background consists of more than ten years of claims processing, medical billing and hospital administration experience.

In addition to overseeing the extensive billing practice, Claudia has provided national seminars in numerous states on Medical Billing as well as training physicians and their staff in several states. You can find her on Prodigy where she is the Careers Bulletin Board Leader and is very active in the medical billing forum.

Your Key To Maximum Reimbursement

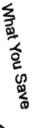

What You Save — What We Offer

⇨ Training new office staff

⇨ Lower overhead

⇨ Postage

⇨ Excessive phone charges

⇨ Stationery and envelopes

⇨ HCFA forms

⇨ Employee vacation, sick, personal time

⇨ Seminar fee's to keep up on the latest changes

⇨ Clearinghouse fee's

⇨ Software and support contract fee's

⇨ Improved cash flow

⇨ Under 3% r rejection rate

⇨ Collections

⇨ Follow-up on unpaid claims and patient billing

⇨ Monthly patient statements

⇨ Daily posting of charges and payments

⇨ Secondary & tertiary insurance billing

⇨ Aging reports

⇨ Referral reports

⇨ Eligibility and benefit verification

~ We Specialize ~

We know rules change for the coverage and reimbursement environment that effect billing.

~ We keep up on the latest ~

⇨ We receive action alerts on the latest changes!

⇨ We know how to bundle codes for higher reimbursement!

⇨ We fight the insurance companies for your money!

~ Our state-of-the-art software ~

⇨ Tracks office visits, capitation, pre-authorizations, prescriptions and certificate of medical necessity.

⇨ Edits the claim before the claim goes to the clearinghouse for a second edit

We attend national and local seminars and conferences to keep up to date.

Our staff is certified through the National Association of Claims Professionals.

We are members of the International Billers Association.

CHAPTER 15

LETTERS, FLYERS & OTHER MARKETING TECHNIQUES

Mailing out a letter with a brochure or flyer is a matter of personal preference. It is hard to determine which is more effective – brochure, brochure and letter, or flyer.

TRUE STORY –

I sent out a Christmas flyer to about 700 doctors. I had used the holiday paper you find in Staples or Office Max during that time of year. Not one response was received which was quite discouraging. About eight months later I received a call from a physical therapist office interested in outsourcing their commercial claims and wanted information. They had filed my Christmas flyer. Needless to say, although we get discouraged when we don't get a response, many doctors/office managers do file away information for later use or "just in case."

Again, let me reiterate to you that this business takes time, and sometimes it takes a lot of time. My word of advice is be patient, be persistent and eventually you will be successful. I have had a lot of discouraging moments. Unfortunately there is no magic formula. Just be patient and let it happen.

The following are various samples of marketing letters. Design your own, you may want to add to the samples I have given. When I started out I enclosed a brochure with my letters. I never received a response from the letters, but my good friend Beverly in California landed four doctors this way.

OFFERING "TWO WEEK FREE TRIALS"

A free trial offer is when you offer the physicians office the opportunity to allow you to file claims for two weeks, 30 days, or a time frame you feel appropriate. The reason people offer a free trial to perspective physicians is to show them the advantages of electronic claim submission in hopes of securing the account. It is also a way for you to get your feet wet if you have no experience. Some people have even used "free claim submission" to find out how the physician office operates, if they are organized and if you really want to have their account.

A two-week free trial will not give a physician's office enough time to reap the benefits of electronic claims submission unless you sign up with a clearinghouse or go Medicare direct. You need to remember and tell the physicians office that a free trial cannot start until you sign up with a clearinghouse. The sign up process takes anywhere from 2-4 weeks, possibly longer. The clearinghouse needs to process your paperwork and get you approved to file electronically. Once that is in place, you can offer this free trial.

There are pros and cons about a free trial. I have heard people who have successfully landed an account that way and I have heard from others who have, at the end of the free trial, had the physician tell them they are not interested. If you chose to go this route, limit the amount of claims you will file. Remember your time is worth money. Don't let a physician's office use you and pick your brain for knowledge.

XYZ BILLING SERVICE

Sally Dodge
President
100 Main Street
Anytown, USA 03030

Telephone 000-000-0000
Fax 000-000-0000

Dear Provider:

XYZ Billing Service is a billing center, privately owned and expanding into your area. My company is comprised of more than ten years of hospital/office administration experience, medical billing, and claims processing.

A successful medical practice provides for patients effectively! Equally important is running your practice as an efficient business. That is why XYZ can help you. XYZ Billing Service will allow your staff to do what they do best by reducing their workload and increasing your cash flow.

Electronic Data Interchange (EDI) has revolutionized the travel and banking industries. Now EDI is revolutionizing the medical industry. Inaccurate insurance filing will be eliminated at a greater saving's than your office staff can accomplish. There will be no more overlooked claims!

YOU CAN SAVE MONEY
AND MAKE MORE MONEY,
AT NO ADDITIONAL COST!

I would very much like to meet with you, or your office administrator, and explain how I can provide these services. At the same time I will be able to explain how the insurance companies are getting interest on your money when you should be collecting the interest.

I appreciate the time you took to read this and look forward to hearing from you. If you have any additional questions or need further information, please do not hesitate to contact me.

Sincerely,

Sally Dodge
President
XYZ Billing Service

OR YOU COULD TRY A SURVEY LETTER LIKE THIS:

Dear Provider:

I would like to offer medical electronic claims processing in the area. I would appreciate a few minutes of your time by asking you to participate in this survey.

Please fill out the questionnaire and return it to us in the enclosed self-addressed stamped envelope.

How many medical insurance claims does your practice process on a weekly basis?

( ) Less than 25   ( ) 25-50   ( ) 50-100   ( ) 100+

In your estimation, how much do you think processing each medical claim costs you?

( ) $4 - $5   ( ) $6 - $ 8   ( ) $9 - $10   ( ) unknown

What is the length of time it takes you to receive payment from the insurance company?

( ) Less than 1 month ( ) 1-3 months   ( ) 3-6 months

Have you investigated electronic claims processing?
( ) Yes   ( ) No

Do you currently process any claims electronically?
( ) Yes   ( ) No

If electronic processing were offered to you, and it cut down considerably on your wait time and total expenses to process medical claims forms, would you consider using it?
( ) Yes   ( ) No

THANK YOU for taking the time to answer our survey. Should you desire additional information by mail on the Electronic Claims Processing System that we will soon be offering in your area, please provide a contact name and a phone number. If you do not wish to receive information at this time, you may leave the area blank.

DOCTOR NAME _____

CONTACT NAME _____

PHONE # _____

ADDRESS _____

CITY _____ STATE _____

Sincerely,

Sally Dodge
President
XYZ Billing Service
1-000-123-4567

Claudia A. Yalden

HERE IS A GOOD EXAMPLE OF A MEETING
CONFIRMATION LETTER. IT ALSO SERVES AS A
REMINDER OF YOUR MEETING.

XYZ Billing Service
100 Main Street
Anytown, USA 00000-1234

Dear Dr. Right:

Thank you for agreeing to meet with me on (day & date) at (time).

In order to prepare for our meeting, please fill out the following information and mail or fax back to me at your earliest convenience. This questionnaire is designed to determine if electronic claims submission would be appropriate for your office and to determine the cost-effectiveness for you to outsource your billing. You are in no way obligated to use our services by filling out this form.

1) How many employees work full-time in the office tending to phones, billing, etc.?

2) How many employees work part-time in the office?

3) Approximately how many patients do you see each month?

4) Approximately how many medical insurance claim forms do you process weekly?

5) How much time do you feel is consumed processing medical claim forms?

6) How much is the average claim?

7) What is your turnaround time on receiving payment from the insurance companies?

8) Do you feel some of your claims are uncollectable? If so what percentage?

9) Does you staff follow-up <u>monthly</u> on unpaid claims?

Any additional information you feel I need before our meeting, please list here:

_____

_____

_____

Thank you for taking the time to send this form back to me. I look forward to meeting you.

Sincerely,

Sally Dodge
XYZ Billing Service

A Survey Letter Which Could Be Mailed With A Brochure

XYZ BILLING CENTER
210 Main Street
Anytown, USA 00000
1-800-800-80000

Dear Provider:

XYZ Billing Center is sending this questionnaire to all area physicians to find out if there is a need for claims to be filed electronically. Please take a moment and answer the following questions. All answers will be kept confidential. This does not, in any way, obligate you to use our services.

1) Does your practice use a computer?

2) Do you process insurance claims for your patients?

3) Are your insurance claims electronically submitted?

4) How many people do you employ (this does not include any professional staff)?

5) How many patients are in your care?

6) What is your estimation of the amount of claims filed weekly?

7) What do you think the time frame is in receiving money from the insurance companies?

8) What is your estimation of claims that are returned because of errors/omissions?

9) What percentage of your receivable do you consider uncollectable?

Any additional information you would like to share, please write here:

_____

_____

_____

Practice Name: _____

Phone # (optional): _____

Practice Contact:

Address: _____

City: _____ State:_____

Thank you for your time.

Sincerely,

Sally Dodge
President

SAMPLE DIRECT MAIL LETTER

XYZ BILLING SERVICE
Sally Dodge, President
100 Main Street
Anytown, USA 03030

Telephone 000-000-0000
Fax 000-000-0000

Dear Physician:

I would like to introduce you to XYZ Billing Service. Our speciality is submitting claims electronically directly to the clearinghouse. By doing this, claims are immediately edited for errors and forwarded to the over 2,500 insurance carriers across the country. We do this using MediSoft, the most advanced, up-to-date specialized full patient accounting medical software. Using our service will help your staff reduce their workload, end the agonizing task of filing medical insurance claims, and allow them more time to follow up on your patients. The result is a higher cash flow in your pocket.

Using our service you would:

- see improved cash flow (direct payment in 18-21 days directly to you)
- know that your claims are being submitted overnight with a confirmation of claim acceptance
- see reduced paperwork
- lower your overhead

XYZ is confident you will benefit from allowing us to process your claims electronically. We are offering a 30-DAY FREE TRIAL OFFER! You can receive an entire month's worth of electronic claims submission on us. If at the end of 30-days, if you are not satisfied, you will be under NO OBLIGATION to continue.

Call us today for a free consultation or to start your free trial. You'll be glad you did.

Sincerely,

Sally Dodge
President
XYZ Billing Service

NOTE: You may want to limit the amount of free claims you are offering.

Claudia A. Yalden

Sally Dodge, President
100 Main Street
Anytown, USA 03030

Telephone 000-123-4568

Dr. Mike A'Phone
33 Cellular Way
Phone Bill Center, USA

Dear Dr. A'Phone:

Electronic claims processing is the future. As you're aware, Medicare has been trying to make filing of claims mandatory. XYZ Billing Service can help you file your claims, and at the same time improve your cash flow. We can give you overnight confirmation on your claims being submitted, reduce your error rate, lower your overhead, reduce paperwork, and have your checks sent <u>DIRECTLY</u> to you.

For a limited time only try our Introductory Free Trial

We will submit your *Medicare/Medicaid claims free for 60 days at absolutely no cost to you. You will be under no obligation to continue if you are not absolutely satisfied.

I would like to stop by and give you a written cost comparison. Please call me today and we can schedule an appointment.

Sincerely,

Sally Dodge

* Offer limited to 25 Medicare/Medicaid claims a day. Subject to acceptance by Medicare and does not include any resubmission because of office error. Offer expires on _____.

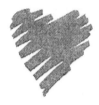

XYZ BILLING SERVICE

Sally Dodge
1100 Main Street
Anytown, USA 00000

Telephone 123-456-7890
Fax 123-456-7899

Dear Dr. Casey:

XYZ Billing Center expanded in your area. If you are submitting claims manually, we can help you. All claims submitted electronically are paid faster (usually within 18-21 days) as compared to a paper claim which has a floor time of 28 days.

We are committed to helping physicians get their money quickly. Right now the insurance companies are getting interest on your money! Shouldn't you be getting that interest? XYZ can provide you with:

- Improved cash flow (the money goes directly to you and payment is made in 18-21 days);

- Confirmation of your accepted/rejected claims;

- Reduced error rate;

- Reduced paperwork;

- Lower your overhead

XYZ would like to give you a "free cost analysis" and discuss the advantageous of electronic claims submission. Please contact us at your earliest convenience, and we would be happy to discuss the benefits of filing claims electronically.

Sincerely,

Sally Dodge
XYZ Billing Service

XYZ BILLING CENTER
Sally Dodge, 100 Main Street
Anytown, USA 00000

Telephone 000-123-4567
Fax 000-123-4890

Dr. Poor Cashflow
777 Money Green Street
Poor Bank Account, USA

Dear Dr. Poor Cashflow:

30-40% of all insurance claims filed contains errors. XYZ Billing Center can help cut through the red tape and file your claims with a 97% accuracy rate. You will see your claims paid in 18-21 days.

We submit claims directly to the clearinghouse where they are edited and sent to over 2,500 insurance carriers nationwide. The clearinghouse also notifies us of any errors or omissions. This means we can correct the claim and send it right back for resubmission.

XYZ has state-of-the-art computers and software to remove the headaches of filing insurance claims. We are able to give you management reports, insurance analysis reports, and a patient receivable ledger report which will help greatly in your cash flow.

Please call XYZ for a "free cost analysis" and let us explain how we can save you time and money. Our fee's are competitive, and we will work hard to see that you get interest on your money. Why should the insurance company collect the interest?

We are available at your convenience to discuss our services. I look forward to hearing from you.

Sincerely,

Sally Dodge
XYZ Billing Center

XYZ BILLING SERVICE

Sally Dodge
President
100 Main Street
Anytown, USA 00000

Telephone 800-123-1234
Fax 800-123-1233

FREE

ELECTRONIC CLAIMS SUBMISSION

FOR TWO WEEKS!

Dear Provider:

Let XYZ submit your claims electronically for two full weeks. Did you know using a medical claim processing service would reduce paperwork, errors, and tremendously improve your cash flow? Right now the insurance company is getting interest on your money . . . why shouldn't you get that interest? XYZ is offering a free trail to allow you the opportunity of benefiting from the advantages of our services.

Your staff can now have the time to follow up on patients rather than have the headache of filing insurance claims. We are trained experts in the field of electronic claims submission and by utilizing our service we can make a difference in your cash flow.

We will process your claims within 24 hours directly to a clearinghouse and you will be able to see a reduced rejection rate. Our clearinghouse directly sends your claims to over 2,500 insurance carriers nationwide.

This **RISK-FREE, NO OBLIGATION OPPORTUNITY** will allow you the opportunity to benefit from the state of the art electronic claim submission process. If, at the end of the two weeks, you are not completely satisfied, you owe us nothing. If you are happy with what you see, we will show you how inexpensive it is to have us file your claims electronically.

Either way, **THIS IS A NO RISK OFFER**, which will expire on **MMDDYY**. We look forward to speaking with you.

Sincerely,

Sally Dodge

NOTE: You need to *be prepared* and have the papers from the clearinghouse ready for the physician to sign. *You cannot sign on to a clearinghouse without a provider identification number.* This process takes approximately two to six weeks. Once the clearinghouse approves the provider the trial offer can begin.

CHAPTER 16

PACKETS AND WHAT TO INCLUDE

SENDING A PACKET IN THE MAIL

The simplest and most inexpensive way to get a packet together for your perspective physician is to type your presentation on your computer, copy it at the local office supply store, and then buy folders that have pockets on both sides. You can probably get 6 folders for a dollar. The folders also have a slit for your business card to be inserted.

You can put a cover letter along with your brochure on one side and use the other side for other handouts that you choose to send. You can also call NEIC (800-877-0004) and inquire if they still carry their brochure (#59450.0PG) which is a colorful brochure listing many of the larger insurance companies who accept electronic claims.

To prepare your materials for your packet, you may decide to use or modify some of the example letters or brochures described in this manual. I also suggest reviewing your competitor's materials. It will aid you in developing your own unique marketing packet.

I never quote a **"fee"** in a packet. You cannot accurately price your services until you know how many claims you will submit and how long it will take you.

MY PACKET CONTAINS:

➢ An introduction letter (which will be your first page)

➢ A brief summary of the company

➢ Statistics (statistics speak louder than words)

➢ Cost analysis of filing paper vs. electronic

➢ A recent announcement as to Medicare rules or which electronic claims will be mandatory

➢ A news article that I feel might be of interest

The following pages will give you an example of various pages I might include in the packet.

I only send packets out when I receive a postcard back from the provider requesting information. Possibly you may send a packet out to a provider who you believe is in need of your services.

You may also want to spend extra money and send a packet when you follow the help wanted ads in the newspapers.

AN INTRODUCTION LETTER

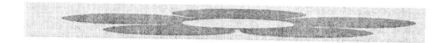

XYZ BILLING SERVICE
Sally Dodge
100 Main Street
Yourtown, USA

Telephone 000-999-8888
Fax 222-333-4444

Dear Dr. Guido:

Thank you for expressing an interest in XYZ Billing Service. I have enclosed information for your review. We are medical billing experts in the Northeast, specializing in electronic claims processing which goes directly to the Clearinghouse. We can:

- Submit claims with a turnaround of 3-14 days, payment in 17-28 days,

- Cut your rejection rate by 33% and,

- Lower your billing costs

Your patients will see how efficient their bills are being handled. They will also be able to reach us at any time to discuss their insurance processing needs.

XYZ can greatly reduce your error rate and improve your collection rate with a drastic reduction in the actual cost of processing. It currently costs you an average of $8 to $12 to file a claim per AMA statistics.

The enclosed information will introduce you to XYZ. We are up on the latest changes relating to the future formats in which a provider will be able to submit claims. Beginning July 1, 1996, HCFA mandated that Medicare can no longer accept claims received in "local formats." The new formats for claims submission are the ANSI 837 and new National Standard Format (NFS). All others will be discontinued.

Let XYZ take the hassle out of billing. Call us at 1-800-123-4567. We will provide you with the personal attention you deserve.

Sincerely,

Sally Dodge

XYZ BILLING SERVICE

Electronic Filing and Practice Management

THE

PRESCRIPTION

TO MANAGING

HEALTH CARE

PRACTICES

OF THE 21st CENTURY

100 Main Street
Anytown, USA 03030
800-000-0000
Fax:800-000-0000

A FACT SHEET ABOUT YOU AND YOUR COMPANY AS WELL AS
THE SERVICES YOU PROVIDE WOULD BE SIMILAR TO THE
FOLLOWING:

XYZ Billing Service

XYZ is a full-service billing center that recently began an aggressive marketing effort due to the recognition by physicians for a need to file claims electronically. The end result is a positive impact on medical practices.

Healthcare has become the largest industry in the United States. The growing senior citizen population is one reason that spending on healthcare is now over approximately $700 billion, and has grown over the last year at an exceptional rate.

Submitting claims directly to a Clearinghouse represents a revolutionary advance within the healthcare and insurance industries.

For both insurers and providers, an excellent opportunity for achieving the goals of better services, cost efficiency, and increasing productivity is modernizing the time consuming task of manually processing paper insurance claims.

XYZ is a full-service billing and insurance claim filing service offering efficient billing to both doctors and patients. With consistent claims submission and the use of electronic claims submission, doctors see their money fast, often within two weeks. Follow-up is the key to steady cash flow and XYZ's intense follow-up procedures is simply unmatched.

Our success depends on your success; therefore, XYZ works hard to maintain a close working relationship with every physician's office. We encourage open communication between our billing staff and the physician's office. By treating our office as an extension of each practice, there is less chance of billing errors or patient problems.

Our fees are customized and based on a percentage or fee per claim basis. There are no hidden costs. The money goes directly to you using your Explanation Of Benefits. We bill you only for what you collect. Our fee's include postage, electronic claims submission, statements and envelopes, claims forms, collection action, management reports, monthly billing to patients, personalized handling of all patient inquires relating to their bills, follow-up with insurance carriers, and an 800 number for your patients to call us.

Our goal is to help you obtain your money as quickly as possible. We are current in federal and state regulations and attend on going seminars relating to the health care industry. XYZ is dedicated to providing your practice with an efficient, cost effective service that can improve your cash flow and build a good patient relationship.

XYZ BILLING SERVICE

PROVIDING . . .

➤ Electronic filing of claims and paper filing when required

➤ Patient, secondary & tertiary billing

➤ Weekly reporting showing all claims submitted

➤ Follow-up on claims submitted for payment

➤ Eligibility and benefit verification

➤ Reconciliation of delinquent accounts receivable

➤ Patient insurance aging report

➤ Practice analysis report (available monthly, semi-annual and annually)

XYZ BILLING SERVICE

Can give you . . .

Submitted Daily Summary - this report informs the provider of how many claims were accepted and rejected by files submitted.

Provider Daily Statistics - this report contains statistics by batch for each provider. Rejected batches and claims are listed with detailed error explanations. It is imperative that this report be reviewed after each transmission to prevent "lost" claims.

Provider Daily Summary - this report is a summary for the number of accepted claims per batch. This report also includes a total section, which displays the number of claims accepted and rejected daily.

Provider Monthly Summary - this report displays the number of accepted claims sent to the receivers including month to date and year to date.

Unprocessed Claims Report - informs the provider that the following claims are unable to be processed by the payor and what corrective action should be taken.

Request for Additional Information - informs the provider that the following claims require additional information for processing. Each message identifies the information required to process the claims and the address to send the information.

Zero Payment Report - will list those claims for which the payor has determined no payment will be made.

INSURANCE PAYMENTS

ARE OFTEN

DELAYED BY:

LOST CLAIMS

REJECTED CLAIMS

MANUAL PROCESSING

CONSTANT CHANGE OF FILING REGULATIONS

WE KEEP UP ON THE LATEST CHANGES AND YOU SEE A FASTER RETURN ON YOUR MONEY!

~ WE WILL ~

WAIVE ALL SET-UP FEES!

ELECTRONICALLY SUBMIT YOUR CLAIMS!

IMPROVE YOUR CASH FLOW!

LOWER YOUR OPERATING COSTS!

REDUCE YOUR CLAIM ERROR RATE!

GIVE YOU A FASTER RETURN ON YOUR MONEY!

~ AND, THE BOTTOM LINE ~

WE HAVE NO HIDDEN FEES!

CONSIDER A FEW STATISTICS:

- Insurance companies and physicians bill over $3 billion dollars annually processing paper claims. Physicians spend over $700 million in postage alone.

- Physicians generate over 3 billion claims each year (that's approximately 95 claims every second of every day).

- Industry average shows that an excess of 33% of insurance claims are suspended or rejected because of paper claim errors.

- Out of the total claims filed in this country annually, less than 10% are being processed electronically.

NATIONAL STATISTICS:

PAPER CLAIMS vs. ELECTRONIC CLAIMS

	PAPER	ELECTRONIC
First-time rejection rate	30%	2%
Payment time	30-90 days	3-21 days
Preparation time	15 minutes	Many < 2 minutes
Cost per claims	$ 8 - $10	$ 2 - $ 4
Advise of problems	After rejection	IMMEDIATE

COST OF FILING A PAPER CLAIM

Assume: 400 claims/month

Cost of Capital	10%
Yearly salary of insurance clerk ((you need to include 25% for benefits)	$ 20,800
Average Claim	$ 50.00
Rejection Rate	30%

* * * * * * * * * *

Insurance Clerk	$ 4.33
Postage	$ 0.33
Forms - HCFA 1500 (.06) - Envelope (.04)	$ 0.10
Cost of Capital	$ 0.62
Rejected Claims Follow-up	$ 0.48
Cost of Capital Rejected Claims	$ 0.13
Billing to Patient (accepted)	$ 1.50
Billing to Patient (rejected)	$ 0.75
TOTAL COST TO FILE A SINGLE CLAIM	**$ 8.23**

CHAPTER 17

THE PRESENTATION

Let me say something about the presentation packet. You marketed the physician. You have already sent them a marketing packet. Assuming they did their homework and read the information, the presentation is the icing on the cake.

If you are nervous you will use your presentation pages as a guide to keep you focused on what you want to say. In my experience, presentations go quickly and you end up in general discussion such as where you are from, your background, experience and other information.

Presentation day is also a day where you will discuss how the claims will be picked up, mailed or faxed! You will discuss your collection policies, your fee, and you will answer any other questions they may have.

You are now at the presentation and like most other people you are nervous. You might fear that the physician would ask you questions that you don't have an answer for. Don't worry! If it does happen, simply tell them that you don't have an answer right now but will have an answer by the following morning.

Presentation day is a day where the physician will meet you and you will flip through your presentation demonstration pages which is a review of the information they already received.

When you get to the presentation you are there to "hopefully" close the deal and negotiate a fee. The physician is now well informed, has met you and should be ready to make a decision to outsource their medical billing.

A True Story –

My first appointment was a result of the post card mailings. I worked in Boston at the time and the appointment was scheduled for a day that I could not take off work. I couldn't cancel the appointment with the physician and I couldn't take off from my job so I talked my husband Bob (who was very supportive) in going in my place which meant that he would be . . . alone.

I briefed him the night before and called him in the morning to give him support on what he should know and elaborated on each page of the presentation package. Bob is not the nervous kind and talking or presenting in a group doesn't bother him. He is in management so he is used to this. However, this time he was nervous but he was willing to help me.

Bob went off to the appointment as if he knew what he was talking about. He apologized to the doctor that I was unable to make the appointment and that he was there on my behalf. Bob flipped through the presentation, describing and commenting to the doctor on information the doctor had already received. When he was finished, the doctor had only a few questions, basically how he would get the claims to us and my collection policy. My husband told him I would get back to him in the morning with the answer. IT WORKED! I had my first doctor and my husband helped me get him.

As far as collection policies go I am asked that question all the time. There are so many laws governing collection and I tell them that right away. I go on to say that I will make calls after thirty or sixty days, sometimes up to ninety days. Then I would give the physician a list and what action I had taken. I let them know it is their decision on how to further handle the accounts. If they want to continue with collections then I would recommend a collection company.

The following pages are some examples that I have used during my presentations. I inserted the pages in a flip chart that you can purchase from any office supply store or from 800-A-PAPERS. I would review these with the physician, much the same way an insurance salesman shows his presentation.

In the beginning when I first started this business I would use all of the pages and there were times when I only used a few of the pages. I feel that the presentation packet is an asset to keep you focused and get your points across.

On Presentation day be prepared with:
✓ Additional information to leave the physician.
✓ A fee schedule providing you had most of the information needed to quote a fee. I am usually prepared with a per claim, percentage and flat fee.
✓ An original contract or agreement to sign.

Questions they will ask are:
✓ How the claims will be sent to you?
✓ When do you bill the physician?
✓ What is your collection policy?
✓ What reports are you going to give them? I always have a sample report with me.

**CLAIMS
SUBMITTED WITH
97% ACCURACY
RATE**

IN OTHER WORDS – THE
CLAIMS ARE MADE PAYABLE
BEFORE THEY ARE
SUBMITTED

 Page 1

LESS COST

NATIONAL AVERAGE
$8 – $10 PER CLAIM

ELECTRONIC SUBMISSION
CAN SAVE YOU UP TO **50%**

 Page 2

LESS TIME . . .

NATIONAL AVERAGE

30-60-90 DAYS

ELECTRONIC SUBMISSION

14-21 DAYS

 Page 3

134

More Money

National Average – Only

Page 4

70% of Claims are Paid

Electronic Submission
Average – 97%

Customized Database

⇒ **Provider Information**
⇒ **Repeat Patient**
⇒ **Insurance Companies**

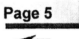
Page 5

We only get this
Information from you once!

Charges Customized
For Your Office

You Only Pay For The Services
You Need

Page 6

We Will Negotiate

"No One Is Too Big Or Too Small"

135

Someday all healthcare claims
will be
processed electronically.

It will save you time & money.

Shouldn't you start saving that
time & money today?

The money you save is yours,
not the insurance company's.
Invest your savings
in your future."

Page 7

Info Needed From The Physician

- New and updated patient and insurance information (superbill or equivalent)
- Insurance company name, policy and group number
- Diagnosis and Procedure codes for each charge
- Physicians fees for each service
- Any correspondence regarding billing or claim submission

Page 8

NOTE: Superbills may be faxed or mailed, unless other arrangements are made.

ADDITIONAL PAGES YOU MAY WANT TO ADD.

~ THE CLEARINGHOUSE ~

WE SUBMIT DIRECTLY TO THE CLEARINGHOUSE WHICH:

➤ RETRIEVES ALL INFORMATION WITHIN **24** HOURS VIA MODEM -

➤ SORT, VALIDATE AND CHECKS AGAINST UPDATED EDITING CRITERIA -

➤ REPORTS ANY ERRORS TO US WITHIN **24** HOURS -

➤ WILL PROCESS AND TRANSMIT TO INSURANCE CARRIERS FOR PAYMENT-

➤ PAYMENT MADE TO THE PHSYCIAN WITHIN **14-21** DAYS -

~ BENEFITS ~

ELECTRONIC FILING WILL REVOLUTIONIZE YOUR CLAIM SUBMISSION PRACTICE BY:

➢ INCREASING YOUR CASH FLOW WITH FASTER PAYMENT OF CLAIMS

➢ ELIMINATING COSTLY CLAIM ERRORS WITH COMPUTERIZED CHECKING OF CLAIMS

➢ REDUCING YOUR REJECTION/DENIAL RATE WITH ELIGIBILITY AND BENEFIT VERIFICATION

BY TAKING THE HEADACHE OF INSURANCE CLAIM SUBMISSION OUT OF THE OFFICE, YOUR STAFF WILL HAVE MORE TIME TO CONCENTRATE ON YOUR PATIENT'S NEEDS AND PROVIDE QUALITY CARE.

CHAPTER 18

CONTRACTS, AGREEMENTS, & FORMS

You will talk to many people about contracts and you will get many different opinions. A contract is a binding agreement between you and the physician. It also guarantees your relationship and the determined fee with the physician for a specified period of time. In recent years I stayed away from the word contract and use the word agreement. Somehow I think agreement is less intimidating.

An agreement can be for any period of time you agree upon. What happens if you decide you don't want to do business with the physician or practice after a few months? Can you void out the contract or agreement? You probably wouldn't want the hassle of going to court to void a contract or agreement, whereby he could easily take you to court for breaking the contract or agreement.

My opinion has changed greatly regarding contracts and agreements. When I first began this business I did not use a contract. My thoughts were if I am doing a good job, and the doctor is happy with me I don't have anything to worry about. I also felt that if I were not happy with the physician or their office staff I wouldn't want to be locked into a binding agreement. Ideally you are looking for mutual benefits and satisfaction.

My thoughts have changed since then on the subject of contracts or agreement. I think contracts or agreements are something you have to really think about. I use an agreement now. I have a clause that states either party can terminate the agreement in thirty days. I am not afraid of losing a practice nor am I going to lock myself in with a practice for a year that I don't particularly care for. There are many people who disagree with my thoughts on this matter however it has worked for me in the past, is working for me now and I will continue doing business this way.

TRUE STORY –

An internal medicine physician called me and basically interviewed me on the phone. We had a great conversation. Since both of us were from New York we talked about the difference in cultures between New York and New England. He asked if I could come up that week and meet. Basically he said "let's get going." Before I left the house that day I knew the account was mine.

His practice has roughly 1500 patients. This meeting occurred right before Christmas so during Christmas week I drove an hour and a half each way to his office for three days and copied all his ledger cards so I could input the data in my computer. He was on vacation so I had the office to myself.

After the cards were copied then came the tedious job of entering the data in my medical billing software. I did not record all the dates of service prior to my taking over the account. I just carried forward his patient balances. I was ready to begin filing claims for him by the first of the year and was really excited about having the opportunity to have my first big account.

Only - I didn't get the account. This situation will not happen to everyone but it should serve as a lesson learned. This particular doctor lost his hospital privileges and was having a nervous breakdown. His wife, the office manager, decided to hold off on allowing me to submit claims electronically. Talk about total shock! Everything you can name is what I was feeling. Not only were my hopes diminished but I also gave up my whole Christmas holiday working on this account.

As of this writing, I don't know whether or not I will ever get the account. I don't really know if I want it anymore. This incident happened over five years ago. I still keep in touch with the secretary every six months or so to keep my name out there. They are still filing on paper. Should the time come when they are forced to file electronically or would like to utilize my services I will decide then or give it to one of my trainee's in the area.

The bottom line when I look back on this experience, I learned a really good lesson. This lesson cost me over 80 hours in time. Had I had a contract or agreement in place at the time then I could have billed the physician for my time.

In the future, when I negotiate with a doctor I will be specific. If the practice is really small I will not have a set-up fee; however, if it is big I surely will have a set-up fee. The set-up fee will cover me in the event I don't submit the physician's claims because they changed their minds.

Many billing centers charge a set-up fee for entering patient data regardless. That is something only you can decide. I will consider each practice as it comes and make my determination from there.

EXAMPLE OF A SERVICE AGREEMENT -

This agreement is made by and between (Billing Center) and (Physician) on the _____ day of _____, 1999.

The parties hereto agree to the following:

1.   (Billing Center) agrees to submit claims electronically for (Provider) or drop to paper when needed within 48 hours after receipt.

2.   (Billing Center) will provide a monthly report to (Provider) on status of his/her accounts.

3.   (Billing Center) agrees that no collection action will be taken unless discussed with Provider.

4.   (Billing Center) agrees to waive all set-up fee's; however, in the event that   (Billing Center) inputs all patient data from (Provider) and (Provider) voids this contract, (Provider) is responsible for the hourly rate which (Billing Center) consumed from imputing patient data, not to exceed $500.

5.   (Provider) agree to pay _____percent/dollars for (Billing Center) fee's monthly. Payment of these charges shall be due within ten (10) days upon receipt of invoice. These rates may change after one year.

6.   The term of this agreement shall be for one year and shall be automatically renewed for an additional year at the date of expiration. (Billing Center) and (Provider) agree that either party upon submission of a thirty- (30) day written notice may terminate this agreement.

_____

(Billing Center)   (Provider)

EXAMPLE OF ANOTHER SERVICE AGREEMENT

This agreement is made by and between XYZ Billing Center, an electronic medical claims billing center, located in Port Jefferson, New York and Dr. Guido on this 21st day of June 1999.

The parties hereto agree to the following:

1. XYZ Billing Center will pick up claims information from provider (or the provider will mail/fax claims) every Friday unless other arrangements have been made, and both parties have agreed.

2. XYZ Billing Center will provide audit entry information from submitted claims to the provider following initial pick-up, unless other arrangements have been made and both parties have agreed.

3. Dr Guido agrees to pay eight and a half percent of monies received from claims submission. Dr. Guido will be billed on the 10th day of each month. Payment of these charges shall be due within ten (10) days. These rates may change at the date of Dr. Guido's annual review.

4. The term of this Agreement shall be for one (1) year and shall be automatically renewed for an additional year at the date of expiration. XYZ Billing Center and Dr. Guido agree that either party upon submission of a thirty- (30) day written notice may terminate this Agreement.

XYZ Billing Center   Dr. Guido
By _____   By_____

SERVICE AGREEMENT

This agreement is made by and between **XYZ Billing Center** and Dr. Guido on this 8th day of June 1999.

WHEREAS, XYZ Billing Center offers electronic medical claims processing services to businesses in the health care industry, and

WHEREAS Dr. Guido wishes to realize increased savings and efficiency through use of XYZ Billing Center's electronic medical claims process services,

The parties hereto agree as follows:

1.0 CLAIMS PROCESSING SERVICES

1.1 **XYZ Billing Center** will pick up claims information from Dr. Guido.

1.2 **XYZ Billing Center** will electronically process and submit Dr. Guido's claims to the corresponding insurance companies and provide a computer-generated report verifying their receipt by the insurance companies. The claims will be processed within two business days, excluding those claims that contain errors.

1.3 **XYZ Billing Center** or Clearinghouse will process those claims that cannot be transmitted electronically and mail them to the corresponding insurance companies.

2.0   COMPENSATION

2.1   Dr. Guido agrees to pay **XYZ Billing Center** for the services described in Section 1 at the rate of 9% of the total claims submitted monthly. XYZ Billing Center will invoice provider at the beginning of each month for the previous month and attach to the invoice a confirmation report from the respective insurance companies. Remittance of these charges will be due in full within 10 days.

3.0   TERMS of AGREEMENT

3.1   Either party upon the submission of a thirty- (30) days written notice to the other party may terminate this agreement.

These parties hereto have executed this Agreement this day and year first written above.

_____   _____
XYZ Billing Center   Date   Dr. Guido   Date

Physician/Patient Information Sheets

The following pages are examples of a Physician Information and Patient Information sheet. You may need to adjust them for your specific needs. The Physician sheet will save you time when you have all the information at your finger tips.

Today physicians have so many identification numbers and you need to be sure you have each and every identification number and that the information is correct. How many physicians that do not know their numbers would amaze you. I have had practices where I have had to call each insurance company to verify the numbers were correct.

The Patient Information sheet is used if you are signing on a new physician, a physician who currently has no forms in their office, or a practice that needs a new updated form.

I find most doctors have some sort of a Patient Information sheet in their office already in place. If the sheet they are using is illegible or has been copied over and over, you may suggest retyping the sheet to give them a fresh original to copy from. Don't try to change what they already have in place unless the information you need is not on the form.

Make sure that the physician has a **"signature on file"** form signed for each patient in his office files. It is critical in case of an audit as well as when you are filing insurance claims. There are two boxes on the HCFA form, box 12 and 13, where the patient should sign and the physician office should keep a copy of the HCFA 1500 in the patient's file.

In your software there is place where you indicate if a signature is on file that would fill in box 12 and 13 on the HCFA 1500 form. Knowing that the physician has his records in order and maintains an up to date "**signature on file**" system for each patient you are protecting yourself as well as the practice.

This is one area I always bring up during a presentation. I will ask the physician point blank - do they have a signature on file or do they use the patient information sheet that the patient signed as "**signature on file?**" If they use the patient information sheet, I suggest to them that they give each new and old patient a blank HCFA form when the patient comes in the office and have the patient sign the blank HCFA form for them to keep in the patient's file.

This should be done in a physician office every year. I suggest to the physician that they get in the practice at the beginning of every year to have their patients update their patient information sheets and sign a new HCFA form.

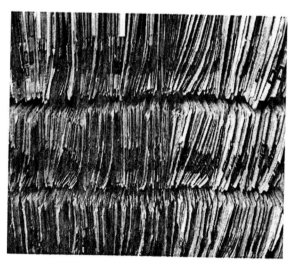

PHYSICIAN INFORMATION SHEET

Have a separate sheet for each physician if there is more than one.

Practice Name _____

Address:_____

City: _____State:_____ Zip: _____

Phone # _____Fax # _____

E-mail (if applicable) _____

Physician Name _____

Office Contact Person_____

Federal Tax ID/SS #_____UPIN # _____

Medicare # _____ Medicaid # _____

License # _____ (if applicable)

Blue Cross/Blue Shield # _____

HMO # _____

Group # _____ (if applicable)

* With so many HMOs and other group insurance companies make sure you have an identification number for each insurance company.

PATIENT INFORMATION SHEET

Name_____ DOB _____ Sex _____

Address _____

City _____State _____Zip _____

Home Phone _____ Work Phone_____

Employer _____
Person to contact in case of emergency _____
Relationship_____ Phone _____

Referring Doctor _____Phone _____

INSURANCE INFORMATION

Insurance Name _____ Name of Insured _____

Insurance Address _____ _____

Insurance Telephone Number _____ _____

Insurance Type: Medicare [ ]   Medicaid [ ]   BC/BS [ ]
Workers Comp [ ]   Other [ ]

Policy # _____Group # _____

Have you met your deductible?   Yes [   ]   No [   ]
Do you have a co-payment for office visits? Yes [   ] No [
If yes, how much? _____

Whom may we thank for your visit here today? _____
Thank you for taking the time to complete this information.
All records are strictly confidential.

CHAPTER 19

SOFTWARE AND THEIR COST

HOW MUCH DOES IT COST?
WHERE DO I BUY SOFTWARE?
WHAT KIND OF SOFTWARE DO I BUY?
DO I NEED SOFTWARE?

When I first made the decision to enter the medical billing business my husband felt I should have a doctor lined up before I purchased software. Being impetuous as I am, I wanted software first, doctor second. I reasoned that I could not learn the business fully if I didn't have the software. I still believe in getting the software first. It allows you the opportunity to learn the software, understand the reports available, and practice on your software. When you speak with a physician you are not only selling yourself, but your software as well. I won the argument, spent $4,000, and had my software.

After three months I signed my first physician and it was time to use my software. I did not practice what I preach today which resulted in my spending eight frustrating days trying to learn the software. It was complicated, difficult, and it was not user friendly. I thought I did my homework on buying software but found out I didn't.

The software I purchased did not meet the specifications of Medicaid in New England. To reiterate what I am saying, each region has their own specifications of where they want certain information. In my case it was the pin number of the physician which had to be placed in box 24K on the HCFA 1500 form. My $4,000 software could not do that nor could it be formatted. Now I use MediSoft and am able to format specific claims forms to certain carrier specifications.

I felt defeated before I even began and felt like quitting. I was told the software was user friendly which wasn't the case. I was told it was easy which it was not. The reference manual that came with the software was not even updated. The software salesman (and partner in his own clearinghouse) came and spent two days training. The two days consisted of several hours of software training, marketing, reviewing the manual and several hours of trying to get the software to transmit to his clearinghouse. What did I know!

Since then, I've come a long way and learned that there are a lot of software vendors out there who use the same approach. It is "**Buyer Beware.**"

A True Story -

After two weeks, I submitted my first batch of claims and thought this was great. I finally did it. It heighten my esteem to think I worked my way through this complicated mess. What I didn't know is that the batch sat in this particular clearinghouse and was never tested or submitted to Medicare/ Medicaid.

Finally after 2 months of tears and frustration I called Medicare and found out they were never submitted. I didn't know that this clearinghouse/vendor was not approved in my region and therefore I could not submit my claims electronically. I called my clearinghouse and learned they were using my claims as test claims. No one ever told me. Then I found out that even though they were to be test claims, someone slipped up and FORGOT about my claims. They were never submitted.

The clearinghouse didn't even report back to me any errors on claims submitted like they promised to do. I was at the point now where I had to face my doctor and explain to him why his claims, which I promised him would have a turnaround of 14-21 days, were still not processed after 60 days.

I thought I would go crazy. My mind was racing and I felt like sending everything back to the doctor, never seeing him again and saying good-bye to the business. Yes, I was ready to quit. Only I kept thinking that I couldn't be a quitter, especially with all the money I had invested. I would also have to face my family and friends. I decided I would have to continue forward and endure whatever came along.

Thankfully my doctor was very understanding. We worked out a mutual agreement. I didn't have the heart to charge him until I had the proper software and patient accounting to handle his account the way I had initially promised. I worked his claims for eight months at no cost.

Then came the time to do "Patient Accounting." I tried Lotus, I tried Excel. I even purchased an accounting system. At this point anything anyone suggested I would try. I was very hesitant to buy new software and go through the ordeal again and I didn't have the money to lay out. Finally realization set in and I knew I had to find the money and buy medical software that had patient accounting functions, and to do the entire job properly, I would also need a clearinghouse.

My grandfather was a big philosopher in saying you have to spend money to make money. ***Proper training is the foundation to success - you have to spend money to make money.*** To this day I realize that his philosophy is true. Many people have tried the same method, one type of medical software, another type of accounting system and needless to say they are not compatible. The result is repetitive data entry for the same patient. Take the repetitive data entry and multiply this by a number of patients and you will find out it will take weeks to accomplish. I learned the hard way, as many other medical billing entrepreneurs have experienced, and now are out of business.

Networking on Prodigy was my biggest inspiration. I met Joanne, Bruce and Beverly. Joanne has a successful medical billing center in Massachusetts. With Joanne's help and inspiration she directed me to temporary filing all Medicare/Medicaid electronically for free and send all commercial claims on paper until I had new software. With Joanne's help I was back in business and once again, motivated. Bruce and Beverly taught me MediSoft and told me I could do it.

There are many, and I mean many, software vendors. Again, don't believe everything you hear. You now have to decide if you want to buy software only or do you want training. You don't want to make a mistake. It is your hard-earned money you are spending. The harsh reality is that many of these software companies and vendors don't care about you, just your money. Will they be there to help you with your business? Once you purchase the software or training will you be all alone? Will you be able to call these people back for support or uplifting? Just be *very* careful when you purchase software and whom you purchase it from.

You may need future support! Where will they be? Will they support you? Did you ever buy a computer or appliance and have a problem and call the store back? What did they tell you? Call service! Once they sold you the appliance they were no longer there for you to help you with your problem.

There are companies who offer you software and marketing training for thousands and thousands of dollars. These companies package software that you could buy for $499 or less. They make a nice profit on their packages. The package sounds wonderful, you travel to the west coast, Florida or New York. They may or may not pay for your airfare and hotel. You stay for 2 or 3 days, spend two days training in a hotel or their headquarters and learn marketing. You never sat at a computer, you didn't see the software except maybe on an overhead, and you didn't learn medical billing. What did you learn? If you are going to buy a package, make sure it is not all marketing.

Finally the two or three days are over and you are on your way home. You're excited. You're mind is thinking of the money you are going to make! You are really psyched. You now have time to think and realize you spent $10,000 and came home with software that you could have purchased for $499. What did you know? The marketing brochures were enticing from these companies and elaborately done. You probably received a lot of extras that really don't account for the money you spent. Don't let these marketing packages fool you.

These companies advertise in USA Today, Home Business, Entrepreneur, etc. They have experienced marketing employees who know how to close a deal. Be very careful. If you are going to spend that kind of money make sure that the training you receive is not all marketing. Your training should *include medical billing and software training – hands on.* Buy from someone that is reputable, that is in the medical billing business and that you can trust. These sales people are high pressured and swift talkers. BE AWARE!

When purchasing software, be sure you know how much the support contract is. Who is it with? Find out if the vendor will help support you as well. How long have they been in business? If you are buying a package make sure you are not a number in a large class. Find out if the training will cover the *technical aspect* of medical billing. Will the information you learned in medical billing be transferred to the software so that you get a good understanding of how the software will operate?

I speak to many people everyday that spent the money from the companies like I mentioned. They get their first doctor and are completely lost. They don't know how to read an explanation of benefits, they don't know if they need a modifier and they don't know how to bill the secondary insurance company. It is really sad that all their money went to marketing and they still had no knowledge of medical billing.

When you're ready to buy software or a training package make sure it is from a reputable dealer. Buy from a software vendor who is in the billing business. I find it unbelievable that a salesperson can sell you software and yet they don't use it. Would you buy a computer from a sales person who never used a computer before? Well, software is much the same way. Someone who has used the software and is in medical billing knows it inside and out. They can understand the problems you may encounter, and can give you the support you deserve.

CHAPTER 20

COMMON QUESTIONS & ANSWERS

How much is software?

In some states you can acquire free Medicare/Medicaid software. Other states will charge for using their software. The problem you will encounter using free software is you will not have a patient accounting system or a tracking system to bill your physician.

If you have experience and feel you don't need training you can purchase MediSoft Patient Accounting software from the Academy of Medical Billing (800-221-0488) for $99. Later on you can upgrade to the $499. Advanced Patient Accounting and receive credit on your $99 software. However; if you have no experience and want to succeed in this business I strongly recommend a training package to give you a solid foundation. This is your future and you should invest your money wisely!

When I buy my billing software package, what training might I expect to receive and how long can I receive support from the company?

Some companies will sell you the software and say good-bye. The price you pay has nothing to do with the bottom line. Investigate the various software companies and learn of their reputation, preferably through other users and associations. Check to see if they are members of the Better Business Bureau in their state. As far as continued informational support and software upgrades, get information on various companies reputations.

Once I have my software, must I deal with a Clearinghouse and if so, what is the cost?

The cost will vary. No, you don't have to deal with a Clearinghouse but it is highly advisable. The cost involved would be per claim, new provider sign up and yearly fee. You shouldn't have to buy any additional software. *I also warn people against buying from a company where you have to use their clearinghouse.* You should be able to pick your own clearinghouse.

What other cost is involved?

Besides buying software you need to consider your office expenses that will include marketing material, computer, phones, HCFA paper, etc. You also need to contact clearinghouses and find out what their fee is. You will be spending money once you start this business and hopefully it will all come back to you.

What should I do first to start my business?

Write a marketing plan (and see how much money you can afford to put into marketing). My recommendation would be to get colorful postcards made up and test your market to see what your response is. If you are getting a response and don't have software . . . buy it. I do recommend having the software before you begin to market so that you are familiar with the functions of the accounting system.

Too many people market and have no training or software. The result is they get a call and buy software. They are not familiar with how the software operates or medical billing therefore panic and make mistakes not counting the time it takes to learn the software.

What kind of practices should I target?

My personal opinion is to begin targeting in on chiropractors, podiatry, ambulance companies, and psychiatrists. They generally are not part of a huge group or an HMO/PPO and if they are they may have a practice on the side away from the HMO/PPO. My first podiatry doctor was part of an HMO and had his own private practice. I only billed for his private practice.

The physicians I mentioned tend to have small practices and do their own billing or hire an outside billing center to help them. A larger practice may be too much to handle in the beginning until you have your software and patient accounting down firm. This is my personal opinion only.

Should I spend the money on a seminar?

Absolutely, knowledge is essential. The networking and knowledge you will gain can save you money in the long run.

Should I order books right away?

If you are not familiar with billing I recommend purchasing "Understanding Medical Insurance, A Step-by-Step Guide" by Joanne Rowell as previously mentioned in the reference section. This book will give you general knowledge of insurance forms. You will also need a current ICD 9-CM and CPT book to file claims.

What should I say in my presentation?

You have a presentation package. Use that package and keep it simple. Don't oversell! Don't undersell! You need to keep in mind the doctor already has a lot of information about your service. Make sure you know how you will pick up the claims, what your fee schedule is, and give him a sheet about what he can expect from your office and what you can expect from his office. Have an agreement ready to sign.

Can I bill for a dental office?

Yes, MediSoft carries PractiSoft for dental billing.

Who can I talk to about the business - how can I reach people?

Use your computer, use the internet, Prodigy, CompuServe, America-On-Line. Network . . . network . . . network! A reputable software dealer will give you names of other dealers and especially other entrepreneurs. Do a press release in your local newspapers and try to advertise in the AMA Newsletter in your state.

Is the Business pretty well locked up by most providers being serviced already?

The market is still wide open. Electronic claim submission is the wave of the future. My personal opinion is that it is still a wide open market. We are in the beginning stages with the advent of healthcare reform and new regulations that I believe will require or force providers to file electronically. Bankers and airline companies have already been conducting business electronically for years and eventually the whole medical industry will follow. It saves money and time, causing increased productivity.

How do I advertise?

Word of mouth, referrals, cold calling, marketing with

letters, postcards and brochures. AMA newsletters, local hospitals. The list goes on.

If I don't succeed, can I get a refund?

Most companies offer a 30-day refund policy. Think carefully, is this business for you? Thirty days is not enough time to succeed in this business. If you want instant success you should not investigate medical billing.

Do I need previous experience?

Having no experience is not a factor; however, I strongly recommend training. Of course if you have some business or medical experience, this may be an advantage. The information to succeed is out there as described in this manual and other publications. The will and desire to learn and perseverance are the secrets to most new ventures.

What is the overall cost to start my business?

That depends on what you are budgeting? You need to take into consideration the software costs and marketing. Again, marketing needs to be persistent and consistent and you need to budget and follow your marketing plan consistently every week.

I am planning on retiring, is there an age limit?

Absolutely not! Matter of fact you can probably take the business with you or sell it.

CHAPTER 21

UNDERSTANDING MEDICAL BILLING

LET'S GET TECHNICAL - As simple as it sounds, if you want to get paid for what you do, you have to speak the language. Physicians use a common language of names and terms to communicate with other physicians and with the organizations that reimburse them for the services they perform.

Understanding Medical Billing is an introduction to medical terminology and their meaning. By no means is this a conclusive guide to the technical task of medical billing.

As you get into medical billing I recommend to everyone that they purchase an ICD-9-CM, CPT and HCPCS book to assist them even further.

The first primary coding system, published annually, is the diagnostic reference, International Classification of Diseases, referred to as ICD-9-CM.

Physicians and other health professionals know the second reference, Physicians' Current Procedural Terminology, as CPT that is published annually by the American Medical Association (AMA) and contains codes for services provided.

The third reference is the Health Care Financing Administration (HCFA) Common Procedure Coding

System, commonly called HCPCS (pronounced "hick-picks"). These codes represent medical services and supplies not specifically identified in CPT, including drugs administered by injection and durable medical equipment. Codes in this system are not as widely accepted as an industry standard as are CPT and ICD-9-CM codes, though their use is growing. HCPC information is presented in Chapter 6.

What you read in the following chapters is by no means an inclusive learning into the medical billing field; however, it is a brief overall of medical billing and designed to assist you in beginning your education and learning in the medical billing field. Medical Billing Specialists need to continue the learning process as they progress in the field. With this section I hope you will gain medical billing knowledge and continue your entrepreneurial career in the medical billing industry.

It is not my intention to overwhelm you with this information, however it is essential in understanding medical billing. If you carefully read, take notes and order the CPT, ICD-9 CM and HCPCS books you will be able to put this technical data into perspective.

Good luck and I wish you much success in your new entrepreneurial venture.

Claudia A. Yalden

CHAPTER 22

CLARIFYING THE ALPHABET SOUP OF MANAGED CARE
AND MEDICAL TERMINOLOGY

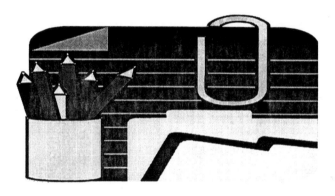

Part of the frustration of dealing with managed care comes from the abundance of new and unfamiliar terms and **ACRONYMS** used to describe it. Here is a handy summary of some terms that will shed some light on what is involved in managed care.

Medigap

Medigap is a secondary insurance, which when filed electronically to Medicare, will be forwarded to the patient's secondary insurance if they are receiving electronic claims submissions.

Managed care

Managed care is an umbrella term for any system that integrates financing and delivery of appropriate medical care by means of:

- Contracts with selected physicians and hospitals that furnish a comprehensive set of health care services to enrolled members, usually for a predetermined monthly premium.
- Has utilization and quality controls that contracting providers agree to accept.
- Provides financial incentives for patients to use providers and facilities associated with the plan.
- Requires assumption of some financial risk by doctors.

Primary Care Physician

A **Primary Care Physician (PCP)** is a patient's primary physician. In a managed care setting a patient cannot go see a specialist unless the **PCP** recommends a specialist. If a patient does decide to see another physician without a recommendation, they are responsible for the payment and chances are the insurance will not pay for it. Most PCPs are family practice, internal medicine, pediatric, and in some plans, gynecology specialist responsible for providing all routine primary health care for the patient.

Gatekeeper

A gatekeeper is a PCP, usually a family physician, general practitioner, internist, osteopath or pediatrician.

HMO's often will not pay for services not approved by gatekeepers, who must authorize medical services, elective hospitalizations, referrals and diagnostic work-ups.

Preferred Provider List

A list of providers with reputations for quality and efficiency compiled by an employer for its employees. These providers have no contracts with the employer and no financial incentives are offered to employees to choose them.

Co-payment

A co-payment is a form of cost sharing in which an HMO member makes a nominal payment to a provider at time of service, typically for office visits and prescription drugs.

Co-insurance

Percentage of cost of care paid by patients as part of insurance coverage.

Case management

Case management is a concurrent evaluation of the necessity, appropriateness of efficiency of services and drugs provided to patients on a case-by-case basis, usually targeted at potentially high-cost cases.

Deductible

A deductible is a set dollar amount a beneficiary must pay toward covered charges before insurance coverage can begin. A deductible is usually renewed annually.

Place of Service (POS)

A Place of Service Code is what insurance carriers use to identify where a service was performed.

POS - Point Of Service Plans

Generally patients do not have to decide how they receive services at the time they originally enroll in a **POS** program. **POS** plans are open panel **HMO** or **PPO** that allows the enrollees to choose between using the network or non-network providers whenever they need medical care. The plan benefits are higher and the patients out of pocket payments are lower if they use a network provider.

PPO - Preferred Provider Organization

PPO is a plan that is not a true **HMO** plan, but they do have more patient care management than is available under regular fee-for-service medical insurance programs. **PPOs** usually do not have contracts for laboratory or pharmacy services, but they do have reduced rate contracts with specific hospitals.

- Most **PPOs** are open-ended plans where the patient accepts a larger out-of-pocket expense if they choose a provider that is not a member of the **PPO**.

- **PPOs** preferred providers have signed contracts to perform services for **PPO** members for specific contract fees. These fees are lower than the fees charged to the provider's regular fee-for-service patients.

- Premiums, deductibles, and co-payments are usually higher than those paid for **HMOs**, but lower than the regular commercial indemnity plans.

Third Party Payor

Third party payor is an insurance company that collects insurance premiums and provides administrative services.

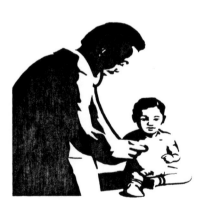

Par Provider (Participating Provider)

A Par healthcare provider is a provider who has entered into a contract with an organization, the government, or an insurance company to provide medical care to enrolled subscribers. In the contract, it is agreed that the health care provider will accept the insurance company's approved fee for each medical service and will bill the subscriber for only the deductible, subscriber co-payments, and any uncovered services as stated in the subscriber's policy.

The benefits of a par provider with Medicare are:

1. Fee's are 5% higher if they participate.
2. Participants are listed in Medicare participating physician and suppliers directory.
3. Participants are provided with a toll free transmission line if they submit electronically.
4. Participants have "one stop" billing for beneficiaries who have non-employment related Medigap coverage.

Non Par (Non Participating Provider)

A Non Participating Provider is a physician that has not agreed to accept the carrier determined, allowed rate as payment in full for covered services performed and, therefore, expects to be paid the full amount of the fees charged for services performed.

PIN (Provider Identification Number)

A PIN is a number assigned to a provider by an insurance company to be used on claims filed by that provider.

UPIN (Unique Provider Identification Number)

A UPIN is assigned by HCFA and given to the physician for purposes of identification on forms and claims.

Superbill/Encounter Form

A superbill/encounter form is the financial record source document used by health care providers and other personnel to record the patient's treated diagnoses and the services rendered to the patent during the current visit.

It will generally contain the patient's name, balance due, date, time, etc. Once the patient is seen the physician will add the procedure and diagnosis that pertain to the visit.

HCFA (Health Care Financing Administration)

HCFA is a federally administrative agency charged with primary responsibility for Medicare and the federal portion of the Medicaid programs.

Purpose of Health Insurance Claim Form – HCFA 1500

The **HCFA-1500** answers the needs of many health insurers. It is the basic form prescribed by **HCFA** for the

Medicare program for claims from physicians and suppliers, except for ambulance services. It has also been adopted by the Office of Civilian Health and Medical Program of the Uniformed Services (CHAMPUS) and has received the approval of the American Medical Association (AMA) Council on Medical Services.

Capitation

Capitation is a fixed payment, in advance, to a provider on a per-member basis regardless of the number of services provided to each member. Rates can be adjusted based on demographics or projected medical cost.

Capitated Payments

Capitated payments are a monthly fee for each patient regardless of the number of times the patient is seen or the type of services performed.

Patient Ledger

A Patient Ledger is the patient account record. It is a permanent record of all financial transactions between the physician and the patients and records the payment or third party payments credited to the patient account.

Fee Schedule

Fee schedule is a predetermined payment from a printed master schedule that sets the maximum dollar amount payable by the insurance company for covered benefits.

A law requires that all copies of the master fee schedule be given to all prospective subscribers at the time they are considering enrolling in a specific plan.

U & C (Usual and Customary)

Usual and customary is a regional average fee profile to determine the "*allowable*" reimbursement for each procedure. U & C is also known as an R&C (Regional/Reasonable and Customary) or **UCR** (Usual, Customary, and Regional/Reasonable) Policy.

Consider the following:

- U&C policies use regional average fee profiles to determine the "**allowable**" reimbursement for each procedure.

- The allowed fee also known as the covered charges for each procedure is established by averaging all the charges for each service submitted to the insurance company by health care provides from a specific geographical region. The allowed fee may be equal to, but never more than, the amount charged by the provider.

- The reimbursement method is updated periodically semi-yearly, yearly, or bi-yearly, depending on company policy; therefore, the reimbursement levels are much more in tune with current fees charged to patients than reimbursement received from the standard, (non-RBRVS) "fee schedule" policies. In return for higher reimbursements, the policyholder will pay a higher premium for a U & C policy.

HMO (Health Maintenance Organization)

An **HMO** is an organized system of care that provides health care services to a defined population for per-person fee. Members are not reimbursed for care that is not provided or authorized by the **HMO**. Think of an **HMO** as a prepaid health care provider group practice servicing a special geographic area.

- **HMO's** are more concerned with promoting wellness. That means they encourage annual physician examinations.

- Some **HMO's** allow walk-in patients who are not members of the **HMO.**

- Some **HMO's** require the patient to pay a small visit charge (co-pay). This visit charge or co-payment will vary according to **HMO** policy, but is normally between $5 and $15 per visit with exception of mental health services, which can run as high as 50 percent if a patient has to be referred outside the **HMO** for this service.

- Most **HMO's** have in-house staff physicians and are paid on a Capitation basis. This means the provider is paid a monthly fee for each patient regardless of the number of times the patient is seen or the type of services performed.

174

(The idea behind Capitation is to provide an incentive for providers to practice preventative medicine in order to avoid unnecessary tests and procedures).

- Insurance forms are not used for processing reimbursement for services rendered to **HMO** patients. The primary care providers within the **HMO** usually see patients. **Remember:** the **HMO** organization is a self-contained program.

- Outside specialists who care for patients referred by their **HMO** primary physician or physicians outside the **HMO** geographical region who see **HMO** patients on an emergency basis will have to bill the **HMO** for services rendered to these patients. This billing can be accomplished using the basic commercial insurance forms.

Rapid growth was seen in HMOs in 1973 with the passing of the federal HMO Act. This act required an employer with 25 or more employees (and who sponsored fee-for-service medical insurance plans) to offer an HMO plan (prepaid contract) as an alternative to the fee-for-service plans.

Fee-for-service

A fee for service plan is a contract in which the carrier pays a set fee or agreed upon percentage of the charge for each covered health care service rendered to a plan enrollee.

IPA (Individual Practice Associations)

- Networks of individual health care providers who join together to provide prepaid health care to individuals and groups who purchase coverage.

- Both **HMO's** and individual employers may contract with an **IPA** for pre-paid, managed health care services for their group members.

- Health care providers in **IPAs** hire their own staffs and ancillary services, such as designated pharmacies, hospitals, and testing labs for all services.

- **IPA** primary care physicians usually are paid on a capitated fee basis whereas **IPA** specialists are usually paid on a negotiated fee-for-service basis that is lower than that charged by specialists to traditional, non **HMO**, or employer group patients.

- These practitioners may also see patients who are not enrolled in an **IPA** program.

SOAP Notes - A charting system

> **S** means subjective impression
> **O** means objective clinical data
> **A** means assessment of the problem and diagnosis
> **P** means plan for treatment, further studies
> and case management

RBRVS (Resource Based Relative Value Scale)

RBRBS is a fee schedule that Medicare adopted in 1991. It considers cost factors involved in all procedures:

- the physician's work factor

- provider's practices expenses less malpractice expense

- the cost of malpractice insurance

Each of these three factors are modified by the geographic index and then multiplied by a conversion factor that is determined annually by the United States Congress which then converts the relative value units into a fee schedule.

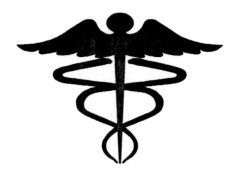

COB (Coordination of Benefits)

A **COB** clause is a contract that is invoked when the subscriber (including **HMO** members) is covered by two or more primary medical insurance policies.

This provision requires that the insurers coordinate the payment of service submitted on the claim so that the patient is reimbursed for no more than 100 percent of their covered expenses.

The primary (principal) carrier pays its full share for covered charges submitted. The secondary (lesser) policies accept the responsibility for the policyholder's deductible, co-payment responsibility, and the insurance company's responsibility for a service that is a benefit of the secondary policy but is excluded by the primary insurance (per the patient's agreement/contract).

This clause prevents the subscriber from being reimbursed two or more times for the same medical expenses. For years, the clause was restricted to group policies where the employer paid at least 50 percent of the premium. In the past few years, many state legislatures have passed state "cost containment" laws making the "coordination of benefits" mandatory for all medical insurance policies in effect within their state boundaries, whether or not the insurance policy specifically states it.

It is always advisable to check with the Insurance Commissioner in yours state to see if a law has been passed to coordinate benefits and how it should be applied.

Rules to follow for deciding the primary and secondary role of a health care policy are as follows:

- **Plan with COB clause vs. plan without COB**

  - *Plan without **COB** is primary.*

- **Plan for active employee vs. plan for retiree**

  - *Plan for active employee is primary.*

- **Plan in patient's own name vs. dependent coverage**

  - *Patients own plan is primary vs. retired plan if involved.*

- **Multiple plans in patient's own name**

  - *Plan held the longest is primary.*

- **Children of parents who are not divorced where both parents are covered by group plans**

  - *Parent with the earliest birthday occurring in the year, not the earliest year of birth, has the primary plan. If the parents have the same birthday, the*

179

plan that originated first is primary. This is often called the Birthday Rule.

- **Children of divorced parents**

    - *Custodial parent plan is primary. If parents are remarried, custodial parent plan is primary, custodial stepparent plan is secondary, and non-custodial parent plan is third.* **Exception: A court order that specifies a particular parent.**

Subrogation

Subrogation is the assumption of an obligation for which another party is primarily liable. Medical insurance policies usually state they will cover "any injury to a subscriber occurring by chance or an error in judgment on the part of the subscriber." The insurance company reserves the right to recover any benefits paid for an injury when the cause or fault of the injury is due to negligence by a third party who has been found liable for the cause of the accident.

EX: *Mr. Jones was injured in a car accident. Mr. Z who was drunk drove the car. Mr. Z did not carry insurance on his car. Mr. Jones' hospital bill was covered by his medical insurance policy. When Mr. Jones won a court suit for damages and lost wages, his medical insurance company asked for and received reimbursement for the money they paid to cover the hospitalization and medical bills.*

The law states that **Medicaid and CHAMPUS/CHAMPVA** must actively pursue subrogation when a third party is liable for personal injuries that have been covered by government sponsored programs.

Clean Claim

The term clean claim means an insurance form that is filled with all data necessary for immediate processing by the insurance carrier. Laws set by the federal government and passed in many states are encouraging insurance carriers to process clean claims promptly. These laws require that interest, generally 1.5% per month, be added to the regular reimbursement for any clean claim not processed within 30 days.

To meet the clean claim standard the following rules apply.

- ✓ Correct spelling of the name of patient and subscriber
- ✓ Correct date of birth, sex, and social security number
- ✓ Correct policy identification numbers
- ✓ Correct name and/or group numbers, if any
- ✓ Correct provider name
- ✓ Correct form (current HCFA form)
- ✓ Correct diagnostic and procedural codes
- ✓ Correct date of service

Procedure

Procedure is the code the physician gives to the insurance company that is a listing of descriptive terms and identifying codes for reporting medical services and procedures. These codes come from the CPT book.

Diagnosis

Diagnosis is the reason the patient is seeing a physician (e.g. appendix, cold, flu, and high blood pressure). The diagnosis comes from the ICD-9-CM book.

Pre-Authorization
Pre-authorization is a number obtained from an insurance carrier authorizing the service(s).

DME (Durable Medical Equipment)

DME is the acronym for Durable Medical Equipment (wheelchairs, commodes, hospital beds, dialysis, etc.).

Medical policies are national in scope (except for regional DMERC policies). Some DMERCs may be slower than others to adopt HCFA policy changes. When there is a discrepancy, follow your DMERC's instructions.

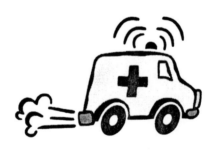

DMERC (Durable Medical Equipment Regional Carrier)

DMERC is the acronym for Durable Medical Equipment Regional Carrier. There are four DMERC regions in the country. They are:

Region A - United Healthcare (Connecticut, Delaware, Maine, Massachusetts, New Hampshire, New Jersey, New York, Pennsylvania, Rhode Island and Vermont)

Region B - AdminaStarFederal, Inc. (District of Columbia, Illinois, Indiana, Maryland, Michigan, Minnesota, Ohio, Virginia, West Virginia, and Wisconsin)

Region C- Palmetto Government Benefits Administrators (Alabama, Arkansas, Colorado, Florida, Georgia, Kentucky, Louisiana, Mississippi, New Mexico, North Carolina, Oklahoma, Puerto Rico, South Carolina, Tennessee, Texas, Virgin Islands)

Region D - CIGNA (Alaska, Arizona, California, Guam, Hawaii, Idaho, Iowa, Kansas, Missouri, Montana, Nebraska, Nevada, North Dakota, Oregon, South Dakota, Utah, Washington, and Wyoming)

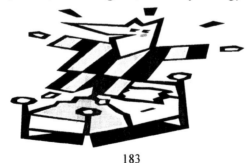

183

EXERCISE

1. Name five key elements for a claim to be designated clean.

    1.
    2.
    3.
    4.
    5.

2. Sally Dodge is covered as a dependent child on two policies. Her mother has a group policy through her employer, IBM. The father has a group policy through the local school district. The father was born on March 23, 1950, the mother on March 9, 1953.

    Who has the primary policy?

3. If the birth date of the subscriber on Policy A was March 13, 1947 and on Policy B it was it was January 21, 1956 which policy is primary?

4. Birth date of policyholder A is 01/21/44. The employee has had group insurance for 14 years, 6 months.

    Birth date of policyholder B is 01/21/44. The employee has had group insurance 10 years.

    Who has the primary insurance?

ANSWERS –

Question 1 -

a) Correct spelling of the name of patient and subscriber
b) Correct date of birth, sex, and social security number
c) Correct policy identification numbers
d) Correct name and/or group numbers, if any
e) Correct provider name
f) Correct form (current HCFA form)
g) Correct diagnostic and procedural codes
h) Correct date of service

Question 2 –

a) Mother born on March 9, 1953 is primary.

Question 3 –

a) Policy B is primary with the earlier birth date.

Question 4 –

a) Policyholder A who has group insurance for 14 years 6 months.

CHAPTER 23

INTRODUCTION INTO THE MEDICAL BILLING INDUSTRY

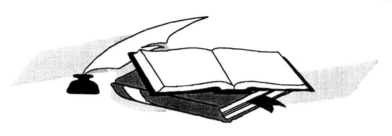

1. TYPES OF INSURANCE POLICIES

The dictionary defines *insurance* as:

> "Protection against risk, loss or ruin by a contract in which an insurer or underwriter guarantees to pay a sum of money to the insured in the event of some contingency such as death, accident or illness, in return for payment of a premium."

Did you know? Over 90 percent of patients seen in a medical office today have some type of insurance policy or other-third party payor.

A ***third party*** payor is an ***individual*** or ***corporation*** that makes a payment but is not a party to the contract that created the obligation/debt.

There are many different types of insurance policies and insurance companies that cover a policyholder including dependent members of their families.

Different types of insurance would include malpractice, automobile, property, life, medical, liability, and disability.

The most common types of insurance are:

1. **Medical:** Various different insurance policies covering the policyholders and dependent member of their families.

2. **Medicare**: A federal program for persons over the age of 65 retired on social security, federal civil service, or railroad retirement and their spouses over the age of 62. It is also for persons who qualify for the federal disability program, end-stage renal disease program, and persons covered over the age of 65 on Medicaid.

3. **Worker's Compensation**: Covers a worker injured on the job who developed a job related illness or injury. It is a program that is federal and state mandated.

4. **Private Insurance**: Private insurance that makes payments for persons who purchased some kind of coverage for private disability insurance and they now meet the qualification for disability.

5. **Liability Insurance**: Liability insurance is generally homeowners or automobile insurance. Liability insurance makes payments for injuries that occurred on, or were caused by some property of an owner, whether it is a homeowner or automobile.

6. **Disability Insurance**: Reimbursement for the lost income resulting from a temporary or permanent illness or injury.

7. **Medicaid**: A program funded by the state and the federal government to provide medical care to those clients who are on public assistance (welfare). It also provides aid to dependent children and certain other medically needy individuals who meet the state's special requirement. (*EX: disabled, obese, mentally retarded*).

8. **Champus:** A federal program for spouses and dependents of persons on active duty in any of the uniformed armed services. It also includes retired personnel from these services and their spouses and dependents.

9. **CHAMPVA:** A federal program for spouses and dependents of veterans with total service connected disabilities that died as a result of service connected disabilities.

TYPE OF INSURANCE PAYMENTS

A.   DIRECT PAYMENTS

Direct payments are payments sent directly from the insurance company to the health care provider's office for payment that was filed on behalf of a policyholder (patient). The check generally covers the third party's obligation (which is the insurance company). The reimbursement will vary from full to partial payment depending on the policy (contract) with the patient.

B.   INDIRECT PAYMENTS

Indirect payments are payments that are sent to the patient as a reimbursement for covered medical expenses incurred. The patient or policyholder has already paid the health care provider.

C.   CAPITATED PAYMENTS

Capitated payments are made to health care providers who are staff members of HMOs where the provider is paid a contractually agreed upon per capita fee for all services provided to an enrollee regardless of the number of visits. Although on-site HMO providers do not use insurance claim forms, some form of internal accounting system is necessary for financial planning.

D.   PATIENT PAYMENTS

Patient payments are payments the policyholder makes to the provider's office whether it is cash, co-pay, or a check.

CHAPTER 24

LEGAL CONSIDERATION

Breach of confidentiality is the unauthorized release of confidential patient information to a third party.

(**EX:** Police officers, government employee's, physician's who do not want information released to their insurance company.)

TO UNDERSTAND BREACH OF CONFIDENTIALLY YOU NEED TO UNDERSTAND THE FOLLOWING:

➢ An **agreement** between two or more parties to perform specific services or duties is called a **contract.** *And,* a third party is one who has no binding interest in a specific contract.

➢ A **contract** is established between the patient and the health care provider when the patient asks a provider to perform medical services in exchange for the patient's agreement to promptly pay the provider's customary fee for the medical services performed. The parties to this contract are the patient, the health care provider and their staff.

191

If the patient is a minor or an incompetent adult, the parents or guardian contracts for the services of the health care provider on behalf of the patient, thus the parents or guardians are a party to the patient health care provider contract.

For providers to properly treat patients:

➢ Patient(s) must be willing to be examined and touched by the medical professions. (*If the patient(s) are to open up to the providers, they must be assured that they can control the release of the information given to the health care providers*).

NOTE: *Breach of confidentiality cannot be charged against a health care provider or their staff, if written permission to release necessary medical information to an insurance company or other third party, has been obtained from the patient or guardian.*

A good maxim to follow is:

When in doubt, have them write it out.

Authorized Release of Information

All medical personnel involved with insurance claims forms should check to be sure the patient has signed an **"Authorization for the Release of Medical Information Statement"** before proceeding to fill out the claim form.

You can achieve this in one of two ways.

1.   The patient signs a **"Release of Medical Information"** block on the HCFA 1500 claim form which is box 12.

2.   The patient signs a special **"Release of Insurance Information"** form tailored to the specific provider's practice that is kept in the patient's chart.

This special authorization form authorizes the processing of claim forms without the patient's signature appearing on each form. The phrase "**signature on file**" must be typed in Block 12 of each HCFA claim form filed for the patient.

A dated, signed release statement is generally accepted to be in force for 1 year from the date stated on the form. A new form must be obtained each year. Undated signed forms are assumed to be in force until revoked by the patient or guardian.

Established practices that do not have a signed "***authorization on file***" for all patients, (but plan to switch to filing claims electronically or to start generating paper claims by computer) must plan to reregister all patients and obtain the necessary ***authorizations.*** This will allow filing claims without the patients signing every claim form.

Two Exceptions to the requirement for having a signed *"authorization for the release of information"* necessary to file an insurance claims are:

1. **Patients who are covered by Medicaid and Worker's Compensation.**

   When a health care provider *agrees* to treat either *a Medicaid or a Worker's Compensation case*, they *agree to accept* the program's *payment as payment in full* for covered procedures rendered to these patients. The patient is billed only for service rendered that are not covered by a specific program.

   The government has stipulated a law, mandating these programs, that the patient is a third party beneficiary to a contract between the *health care provider and the governmental agency* that has responsibility for the program.

2. **Patients who are seen at the hospital.** Filing insurance claims for medical services (provided by a physician) to a patient who is seen at a hospital and who are not expected to receive follow-up care in the physician's office.

   These patients had to sign an *"authorization for treatment and an authorization for release"* of medical information at the hospital before they are seen by the health care provider in the hospital. Should they go to the provider's office another *"authorization for release"* must be on file.

Note: If the hospital's medical information release form is written to include both the release of information from the hospital and the treating physician, claims may be submitted by the physician's office without having to obtain a separate medical information release from the patient. The words *"Signature on file"* are written in the *"Authorization For The Release of Medical Information"* signature block 12 on the medical insurance claims form.

Types of Authorizations

1. Commercial Insurance

2. Medicare Insurance

3. Medicare Supplemental Insurance

4. Authorization for the release of HIV status

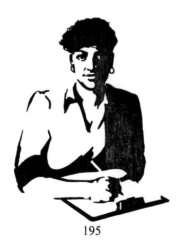

195

TELEPHONE QUERIES

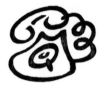

REGARDING CLAIM INFORMATION

Breach of confidentiality can occur when you are asked to clarify insurance data over the phone. Even though you are absolutely **sure** you have a **signed release statement on file** -

> *"CAN YOU be equally sure that the person who placed the phone call is actually entitled to the information?"*

It is easy for a curious individual to place a call to a physician's office and claim to be an insurance company benefits clerk.

Never give information over the phone or in person until you have verified that the party making the request is entitled to the information.

Verify telephone inquiries –

- **PROTECT YOURSELF** - Return the call through the caller's company switchboard.

- Put the caller on hold until you have the file copy of the patient's insurance claim form in hand.
- Ask the caller to read the line of the claim form that needs clarification.
- Follow up this action by writing a detailed memo of the conversation. Make sure you **file this detailed memo along with a copy** of the claim form.

If they need several questions or detailed clarification, have them send you a written request for the information. If verification cannot be made to your satisfaction, ask the caller to put the request in writing on company stationary.

BEWARE of calls from lawyers who request information over the phone. They are well aware you must actually have the patient's signed release of information in hand before answering questions.

Never take the attorney's word that they have a signed release from the patient and do not give in to their request when they say "just answer this little question."

Also, office and billing personnel, or medical assistants who give out confidential information to a person who has no demonstrable need to know is *breaching the confidentially* of a patient.

Remember patient confidentiality is:

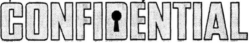

INSURANCE FRAUD AND ABUSE

The Medicaid and Medicare Patient and Program Protection Act of 1987 defines *fraud* as:

"intentional deception or misrepresentation that an individual makes, knowing it to be false which could result in some authorized benefit."

And *insurance abuse:*

"incidents by or providers, physicians, or suppliers of services and equipment which, while not considered fraudulent, are not consistent with accepted sound medical, business or fiscal practices."

EXAMPLE:

- Billing for services that were not rendered - (billing a patient/insurance company for a patient that was scheduled for an appointment but failed to keep.)

- Subsequent billing for excessive and unnecessary care (testing all patients with complaints of sore throat.)

- A health care provider requesting a diagnosis be put on the patient's insurance claim form that is different from the one the provider has written in the patient's chart.

- A heath care provider requesting treatments be added to the insurance claim form that are not in the patient's chart or charge slip or on the patient's account/ledger.

- A health care provider asks you to increase the charges on the insurance claim form by "x" amount because the patient is covered by insurance.

- A patient or provider asks you to change the date of treatment on the ledger/account and the claim form.

- Patients requesting a typed statement of only the charges (w/o insurance payment) of their accounting.

- Patients who ask you to change the date of treatment. (They may not be eligible for coverage on the date treatment was performed.)

- Requests for typed statements detailing only the charges on the account may be an attempt to prove a larger medical deduction on their income tax than patients are entitled to receive or patients may be trying to circumvent a **coordination of benefits clause** in their insurance policies.

Remember The Coordination Of Benefits Clause

*When a patient is covered by two or more medical insurance policies a "**coordination of benefit clause**" will restrict payment by the primary insurance companies to no more than 100 percent of the covered benefits.*

The second insurance company will require a statement of benefits paid by the primary insurer before paying its share of the procedures performed.

PENALTIES FOR FRAUD AND ABUSE

By law, claim forms for government programs (Medicare, Medicaid, CHAMPUS, Worker's Compensation, and the Federal Employees Health Benefit Programs), require that the provider, or their designated agent, sign the claim attesting to the fact that the diagnostic and procedural information supplies on the claim form is accurate.

The penalty for an established pattern of fraud and abuse ranges from criminal or civil conviction through the federal court system to administrative penalties levied by the Office of the Inspector General.

The fines can be as high as $5,000 for each incident.

Non governmental programs also have protection against fraud as established by the individual state's civil courts, although statements warning about fraud are not usually included on the claim form.

When an insurance company suspects fraud they have the right to examine the patient's chart and ledger card

If one case of fraud is found, the insurance company may then ask the court for permission to do a general audit of all claims filed by the health care provider. Many cases of fraud are first detected when:

~ a patient receives an "Explanation of Benefits" (EOB) form from the insurance company that details how benefits were determined for filed claims. ~

When a pattern of fraud is found or suspected, the non-governmental program often notifies the various governmental programs of the suspected problem, thereby enlarging the scope of investigation to include both state and federal statues.

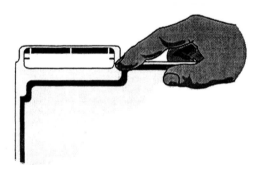

PREVENTION OF FRAUD

Prevention of Fraud is to ensure against becoming inadvertently involved in fraud. It is your responsibility to be sure that all insurance information is true.

- Never honor requests to change information as is stated in the legal records of the patients.

- Never add a diagnosis to an insurance claim that has not first been charted in the patient's chart by the healthcare provider. (If you think a diagnosis has been inadvertently left off the chart, ask the provider to make an addendum in the chart before putting the information on the insurance form.)

- Never add a procedure to an insurance claim form that is not recorded on both the patient's chart and ledger.

When in doubt, have them write it out!

Coding Error Penalty

Civil penalties for misrepresentation of diagnoses and medical treatment are contained in the Omnibus Budget

Reconciliation Act of 1986 and Omnibus Budget Reconciliation Act of 1987 (ORB 1987).

These laws state that physicians can be assessed civil penalties if they:

"know of or should know that claims filed with Medicare or Medicaid on their behalf are not true and accurate representation of the items or services actually provided."

BOTTOM LINE: Providers can be held responsible - **not only for negligent mistakes they make but also for mistakes made in their behalf by insurance specialists or medical assistants.**

These penalties are assessed for $2,000 per violation (a single coding error), an assessment in lieu of damages of up to twice the amount of error on the claim form, and exclusion from Medicare and Medicaid programs for up to 5 years.

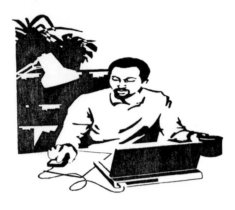

PREVENTION AND CORRECTION OF MISTAKES

- Careful proof reading of the diagnostic and procedures code numbers when data is entered in the computer or on claims forms

- Checking the EOB statement that accompanies all direct payments of insurance claims to be sure that the correct diagnostic and procedure codes were picked up by the key punch operators and entered into the insurance companies' computers or data transfer was complete and accurate when claims are submitted electronically.

  (If the wrong diagnostic and procedure codes show on the EOB form, notify the insurance company (in writing) that an error in processing has occurred. A copy of the original claim form and a copy of the EOB form should accompany the letter.)

CHAPTER 25

LIFE CYCLE OF AN INSURANCE CLAIM

1. An insurance claim begins when the patient makes the call to the physician's office.

2. Patient is established as a new or established patient to the practice.

3. Determine if a managed care program that has authorized the health care provider to perform services covers the patient. All new patients who are enrolled in managed care programs must have prior authorization from their primary care physician or case manager for all services performed by non primary care providers.

Primary care physician (PCP) is a family practice, internal medicine, pediatric, and in some plans, gynecology specialist responsible for providing all routine primary health care for the patient.

Case manager is a nurse, or other medically trained person who coordinates the care of patients with long-term chronic conditions.

---

4. Patient Registration Form is filled out

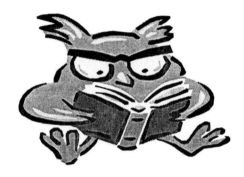

MANAGED CARE AUTHORIZATIONS

It is the patient's responsibility to obtain from the PCP the initial authorization for specialty care of ancillary services. The PCP will give (1) patient a written Primary Care Referral Form. The referral is either hand carried by the patient or faxed to the specialist/ancillary services provider; (2) or a case manager calls the specialist's office to inform the office that a specific patient is being referred to the health care provider and will be calling for an initial appointment.

A POINT TO REMEMBER: Managed care programs not only pre-authorize all services by outside specialist and ancillary providers but also specify the time frame that the authorization is in force. If the number of services is exceeded or the services are performed outside the authorized time frame, payment for services may be disallowed as unauthorized care.

ESTABLISHED PATIENT AUTHORIZATION

Before a managed care established patient receives any services the status of the authorization for care must be checked.

This is usually done 1 or 2 days prior to the patient's appointment for non-emergency care allowing time for the faxing to PCP or case managers for the necessary treatment reports required to re-new authorizations.

Although I have listed the sequence to entering patient data in a physician office, as a billing center you will not be responsible for all the steps but should be aware of the process.

Sequence to entering data

i.   Obtain necessary authorizations.

ii. Fill out the patient encounter form. The encounter form (also known as charge slip) is the financial record source document used by health care providers and other personnel to record the patient's treated diagnoses and the services rendered. The minimum information entered on the form is the date, patient's name, and balance due on the account. The encounter form may vary from a simple blank piece of paper to a rather complex, customized preprinted check off sheet more commonly known as the superbill.

iii. List all services rendered and treated diagnoses on the encounter form.

iv. Price and code all procedures and diagnoses.

v. Enter all procedures, charges, and payments on the daily accounts receivable journal (the daily accounts receivable journal is also known as a day sheet and, is a chronological summary of all transactions posted to individual patient ledgers on a specific day).

vi. Post all charges and payments to the patients account. The patient ledger, also known as the patient account record in a computerized system, is the permanent record of all the financial transactions between the patient and the practice. Posted on this ledger/account are the charges and personal or third party payments credited to the patient's account. Each procedure must be individually described and priced on the ledger/account. The source of each credited payment should be identified, either as cash, personal check, or third-party payment.

vii. Develop the insurance form.

viii. Note the claim completion.

ix. Attached any necessary documentation.

x. Provider signs or stamps.

xi. File copy of the claim form and any attachment sent with the claim.

xii. Record claim in practice's insurance registry.

xiii. Mail claim to the insurance company

xiv. Mail copy of the patient's ledger/account to the patient.

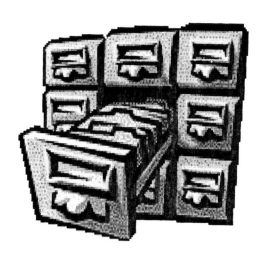

HOW AN INSURANCE COMPANY PROCESSES A CLAIM

1. Claim is computer scanned for patient and policy ID number. If the numbers and/or patients name is wrong the claim is immediately rejected. Claims will also be automatically rejected if the patient and subscriber names do not match exactly with the names on the master policy list. Use of nicknames or typographical errors here will cause rejection and return of the claim to the provider.

2. Procedure codes on the claim are matched with the policy's master benefits list. Any service that is determined as non-covered will be marked as an uncovered procedure and rejected for payment.

3. Procedure codes are cross-matched with diagnostic codes. Services considered to be not "*medically necessary*" will be rejected.

4. Claim is checked against the patient's common data file. A common data file is an abstract of all recent claims filed for that patient. This is a check to determine if the patient is receiving concurrent care for the same condition by more than one provider and to determine if the services are related to recent surgeries, hospitalizations or liability coverage.

5. Determination is made of "*Allowed Charges*."

(Allowed charge is the maximum amount the insurance company will pay for each procedure or service according to patient policy. The amount will vary according to the contract.)

6. Patient's deductible is determined.

7. The co-payment or coinsurance is determined.

The co-payment is a provision in an insurance policy requiring the policyholder to pay a specified percentage of each medical claim.

8. The Explanation of Benefits form is completed.

The EOB is a report or statement that tell the patient or provider how the insurance company have determined its share of the reimbursement. The report includes the following information.

- A list of all procedures and charges submitted on the claim form
- A list of any procedures submitted but not considered a benefit of the policy
- A list of all the allowed charges for each covered procedure
- The amount of the patient deductible if any subtracted from the total allowed charges.
- The patient's financial responsibility for cost-sharing (co-payment) for this claim

- Total amount payable by the insurance company on this claim

9. The Explanation of Benefits and check is mailed.

   If the claims form stated that direct payment should be made to the physician, the reimbursement check and a copy of the EOB will be mailed to the physician. This can be accomplished in one of three ways:

- The patient signs the Authorization of Benefits Statement, Block 13 on the HCFA 1500 form.

- The physician marks "YES" at block 27 on the claim form.

- The physician has signed an agreement with the insurance company for direct payment of all claims.

   If the reimbursement is to be sent to the patient, the policyholder will receive a copy of the EOB, but none is sent to the provider.

The Typical Flow Of A Manual (Paper) Claim

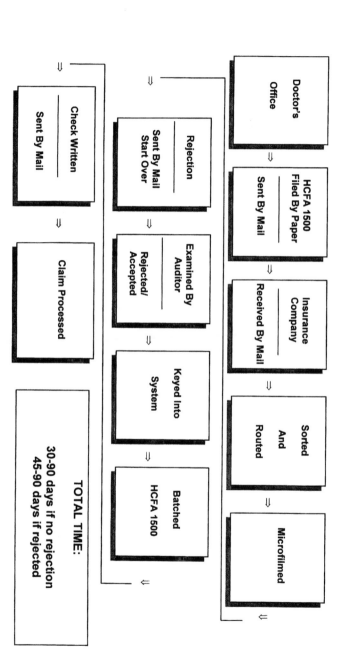

Doctor's Office

⇓

HCFA 1500 Filed By Paper
Sent By Mail

⇓

Insurance Company
Received By Mail

⇓

Sorted And Routed

⇓

Microfilmed

⇓

Batched HCFA 1500

⇓

Keyed Into System

⇓

Examined By Auditor
Rejected/ Accepted

⇓

Rejection
Sent By Mail Start Over

⇓

Check Written
Sent By Mail

⇓

Claim Processed

TOTAL TIME:
30-90 days if no rejection
45-90 days if rejected

CHAPTER 26

THE CPT FORMAT

Before beginning the **CPT** Format section I urge you to order the **CPT** book. Having the book at your side as you read through this chapter will help you in understanding the coding system.

The term **CPT** is an acronym for **Current Procedural Terminology**.

The **CPT** coding system is based on a five-digit main number to describe particular services.

CPT codes and terminology serve a variety of important functions in the field for reporting of physician procedures and services under government and private health insurance programs.

Medicare and Medicaid programs mandate the use of **CPT** codes and with few exceptions, most commercial insurance carriers also use **CPT** codes. Most of the **exceptions** to the use of **CPT** codes are found in the processing of **workers' compensation claims** and in **billing some HMOs**.

The main body of the **CPT** is divided into **six** sections. Within each section are **subsections** with anatomic, procedural, condition, or descriptor subheadings. The procedures and services with their identifying codes are listed in numeric order **except** for codes found in the *EVALUATION AND MANAGEMENT* section (99200-99499).

NOTE: These codes (Evaluation and Management) are located at the beginning of the CPT. They are used by all medical professionals and are the most frequently used codes.

The **CPT** coding system, based on a five-digit main number, describing a particular service may sometimes be used with a *two-digit code modifier* that may be added after the *five-digit* main number.

A two-digit modifier is used when it is necessary to indicate that the service performed deviated from the average service for that specific code number or to specify a particular part of the body.

It should be noted that these CPT modifiers are not presently applied to claims submitted by ambulatory surgical centers or outpatient services filed by institutions.

THE SIX SECTIONS CONTAINED IN THE CPT CODING SYSTEM:

Evaluation and Management	99201 to 99499
Anesthesiology	00100 to 01999
	99100 to 99140
Surgery	10040 to 69990
Radiology	70010 to 79999
Pathology and Laboratory	80049 to 89399
Medicine	90281 to 99199

USING A CPT CODE

The use of a **CPT** code is quite simple. A patient sees a physician for a procedure or service. That procedure or service needs to be coded which means the physicians must identify the service performed using a **CPT** code.

The **CPT** procedure terminology has been developed as stand-alone descriptions of medical procedures. In addition to the **CPT** code a physician may then use a modifier. A modifier will provide the physician the means by which they can further indicate that a service or procedure that has been performed has been altered by some specific circumstance.

Modifiers can obviate the necessity for separate procedure listings that may detail the circumstances. Modifiers are used to indicate:

- ✓ A service or procedure has both a professional and technical component

- ✓ A service or procedure was performed by more than one physician or in more than one location

- ✓ A service or procedure has been increased or reduced

- ✓ Only part of a service was performed

- ✓ A bilateral procedure was performed

- ✓ A service or procedure was provided more than once

- ✓ Unusual events occurred

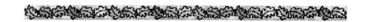

EXAMPLE OF USING A MODIFIER:

1. CPT Code 10060 (Incision and drainage) with modifier –51 (indicating multiple procedures)

2. L8030 (breast prosthesis) with modifier RT (indicating right breast)

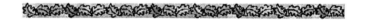

SOME COMMON MODIFIERS ARE:

-21   Prolonged Evaluation and Management Services

-22   Unusual Procedural Service

-23   Unusual Anesthesia

-24   Unrelated Evaluation and Management Service by the Same Physician During a Postoperative Period

-25   Significant, Separately Identifiable Evaluation and Management Service by the Same Physician on the Same Day of the Procedure or Other Service

-50   Bilateral Procedure

-51   Multiple Procedures

-79   Unrelated Procedure or Service by the Same Physician During the Postoperative Period

This listing is by no means conclusive.

Again, I urge everyone to order a CPT, ICD-9 and HCPCS book when they begin this business. To further educate themselves in the use of codes, diagnosis and modifiers I recommend reading the front cover, forward, introduction, appendix(s) and the back cover. There is a wealth of information in those books and through careful study, it is amazing what you can learn.

In addition, listed in every CPT books is a summary of all the code additions, deletions, and revisions. It is an annual update of codes that have been deleted, revised or added. It is necessary to review these codes annually and made any changes in your software to keep current on updated codes

CPT SYMBOLS AND CONVENTIONS

Each book will also have its own symbols, coding and conventions to further clarify their meaning. CPT Symbols and Conventions are used for proper coding of procedures and cannot be accomplished without a thorough understanding of the symbols and conventions used in the coding system. A code such as • would indicate that the code is a new code.

There are some very important symbols that precede a code number. These symbols are used throughout coding books. A few of these are:

▲ The triangle indicates that the code description has been revised from the last annual edition of the CPT.

• The bullet indicates that this is a new code, which appears for the first time in this edition of the code.

* The surgical section uses an asterisk (*).

The (*) will appear after the code number of minor surgery indicating a surgical procedure.

In addition,

;   The semicolon is used to separate the main and subordinate clauses in the code description. This symbol was adopted to save space in the coding books when there is a series of related codes. The main clause will appear in the first description at the beginning of the series and is not repeated in the successive indented codes in the same series.

New subordinate clauses, which differentiate one code from another appears as indented on a new line and usually begin with a lowercase letter.

(The exception to the first word beginning with a lowercase letter is when the subordinate clause begins with an eponym).

As a medical billing specialist you are not responsible for coding. All codes must come from the physician's office. Only a certified coder is allowed to code. This is a field you may eventually want to enter to further your education. Most local community colleges in your area offer coding classes however, since you are a medical billing specialist it is important to know your responsibility is not coding – only taking the information the physicians office has given you.

A certified coder has a lot of responsibilities. Some of them include:

✓ Reading thoroughly the guidelines at the beginning of each CPT section.

✓ Reading carefully each procedure statement listed on the charge slip/encounter slip, operative and laboratory report.

✓ Going to the index to look up the main term in the procedure or service on the source document. This will be one of the following: (1) the action, (2) site, (3) condition, (4) synonyms, and (5), eponyms

✓ Locating any necessary sub-term and follow any cross-reference mentioned in the index.

The code descriptions of all codes listed for the specific procedure or service must be read thoroughly. Remember if the last code description read is at the bottom of the page, turn the page and check to see if the topic is continued.

If an adequate code in the CPT cannot be located research HCPCS Level II and Level III codes. Assign a proper main code number. *(If the code number cannot be found in the CPT Level II and III codes, consult with the physician*.) Assign any modifiers warranted by special circumstances.

SURGERY SECTION OVERVIEW

DEFINITION:

➤ Surgery is considered any treatment that breaks the normal skin such as injections, incisions, and excisions.

➤ Examination with the aid of a scope that goes beyond the normal body.

➤ Treatment for burns.

➤ Treatment for a fracture.

➤ Any procedure fitting the popular definition of surgery.

The surgical section is organized by body systems. Each system is subdivided first by the specific organ or anatomical site and then by broad procedure categories of the following order:

➤ Incision

➤ Destruction

➤ Excision

➤ Introduction

➤ Removal

223

➢ Repair

➢ Endoscopy

➢ Grafts

➢ Suture

➢ Other miscellaneous procedures

In order to code surgeries properly, three questions must be asked:

1. What body system was involved?

2. What anatomical site was involved?

3. What type of procedure was performed?

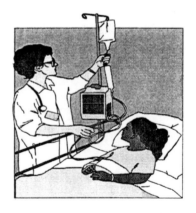

CHAPTER 27

UNDERSTANDING HCPCS

The term **HCPCS** can be confusing. **HCPCS** (*HCFA Common Procedure Coding System*) is most accurately used as the acronym for the entire **three-level HCFA Common Procedure Coding System.** **HCPCS** is also most commonly used to identify **HCPCS** Level II National Codes.

HCPCS are categorized in a three level coding system which incorporate:

➤ **Level I - CPT**

➤ **Level II - National**

➤ **Level III - Local Codes**

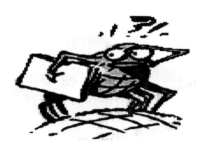

HCPCS codes must be used when billing Medicare carriers and, in some states, Medicaid carriers. Some private insurance carriers also allow or mandate the use of **HCPCS** codes.

The **HCPCS** coding system is used primarily to bill Medicare for supplies, materials, injections and services performed by physicians or other health care professions. Each supply, material, injection or service is identified with a **five-digit** code that begins with an alphanumeric letter followed by four numbers.

Let's put HCPCs in perspective –

Before you apply **HCPC** codes, you need to check for Level III codes assigned by your local Medicare carrier, State Medicare office or private payer. **Level III** codes are used over **Level II** codes, which are used over **Level I** codes.

Before I go on I don't want to completely scare you with the process of using **CPT** and **HCPC** codes. Physicians are the one who will be coding and you will not be responsible for the codes. However, you need to be aware of the difference between **CPT** and **HCPC** codes as well as the different levels of coding which are:

LEVEL I

Level I is the **CPT** that lists the **five digit codes** with descriptive terms for reporting services performed by healthcare providers and is the country's most widely accepted coding reference.

LEVEL II

Level II codes is the **HCPC's** National Codes. *CPT does not contain all the codes needed to report medical services and supplies*, therefore HCFA developed the second level of codes.

These codes begin with a single letter (**A through V**) followed by **four numeric digits**. The service or supply they represent groups them. Unfortunately, an increasing number of private insurance carriers are also encouraging or requiring the use of **HCPC** National Codes which makes this book essential in your library.

LEVEL III

Level III codes are assigned and maintained by individual state Medicare carriers. These codes begin with a letter (**W through Z**) followed by **four numeric digits**. These codes are not common to all carriers. These codes are used to describe new procedures that are not yet available in **Level 1 or II**. These are introduced on an as-needed basis throughout the year.

WHAT IS THE PURPOSE OF THE HCFA COMMON PROCEDURE CODING SYSTEM?

HCPCS is a uniform method for healthcare providers and medical suppliers to report professional services, procedures, and supplies. HCFA developed this system in 1983 to:

➢ Meet the operational needs of Medicare/Medicaid.

➢ Coordinate government programs by uniform application of HCFA policies.

➢ Allow providers and suppliers to communicate their services in a consistent manner.

➢ Ensure the validity of profiles and fee schedules through standardized coding.

➢ Enhance medical education and research by providing a vehicle for local, regional, and national utilization comparison.

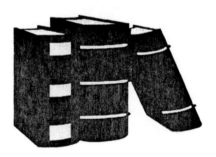

THE THREE MOST COMMON PROBLEMS WHICH ARISE FROM HCPCS CODING ARE:

1. General lack of knowledge and understanding about exactly how and when to use the HCPCS National Level 2 or Local Level 3 codes instead of CPT.

2. Carrier discretion (the use, interpretation and reimbursement policies) for HCPCS National Level 2 codes which should be uniform nationwide, may vary from carrier to carrier.

3. The assignment, use, interruption, reimbursement, and combination of HCPCS Local Level 3 codes and modifiers vary greatly from carrier to carrier.

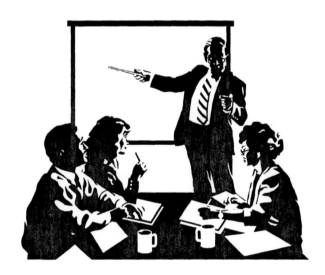

HCPCS LEVEL 1: CPT

As mentioned in the previous chapter, **CPT Level 1** is the major portion of the **HCPCS** coding system. **CPT** codes are five-digit numeric codes. Most of the procedures and services you perform, even to Medicare patients, are billed using **CPT** codes. The major deficiency with the usage of the **CPT** code is that it has <u>limited code selections</u> to describe supplies, materials and injections.

HCPCS LEVEL II – NATIONAL CODES

HCPCS National **Level II** codes are alphanumeric codes that start with a letter followed by four numbers. The range of National **Level II** codes is from **A0000 through V0000**. There are also National **Level II** modifier codes.

National **Level II** codes are uniform in description throughout the United States when describing covered services to Medicare intermediaries. However, due to carrier discretion, the processing and reimbursement of National **Level II** codes is not necessarily uniform.

There are over **2,400 HCPCS** National **Level II** codes covering supplies, materials, injections and services. A fundamental understanding of how and when to use HCPCS National **Level II** or Local **Level III** codes can have a significant impact on your Medicare reimbursement.

The majority of physicians will only use codes from the Medical and Surgical Supplies section and Drugs Administered by Other Than Oral Methods, commonly referred to as "A" codes and "J" codes.

A health care professional using **HCPC** National **Level II** codes selects the name of the material, supply, injection, service or procedure that most accurately identifies the service performed or supply delivered.

Most often, **HCPC** National **Level II** codes will be used instead of, or in addition to **CPT** codes for visits, evaluation and management services, or other procedures, performed at the same time or during the same visit. All services, procedures, supplies, materials and injections should be properly documented in the medical record.

The listing of a supply, material, injection or service and its code number in a specific section of **HCPCS** does not usually restrict its use to a specific profession or specialty group. There are some **HCPC** National **Level II** codes that are by definition, profession or specialty specific.

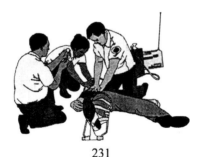

HCPCS LEVEL II CODES

HCPCS Level II codes are divided into twenty sections. The supplies, materials, injections and services are presented in numeric order. The twenty major sections of HCPCS are:

Transportation Services	A0000-A0999
Chiropractic Services	A2000-A2999
Medical and Surgical Supplies	A4000-A4999
Miscellaneous and Experimental	A9000-A9999
Enteral and Parenteral Therapy	B4000-B9999
Dental Procedures	D0000-D9999
Durable Medical Equipment (DME)	E0000-E9999
Procedures/Services Temporary	G0000-G9999
Rehabilitative Services	H5000-H5999
Drugs Administered Other Than Oral Method	J0000 -J8999
Chemotherapy Drugs	J9000-J9999
Temporary Codes For DMERC	K0000-K9999
Orthotic Procedures	L0000-L4999
Prosthetic Procedures	L5000-L9999
Medical Services	M0000-M9999
Pathology and Laboratory	P0000-P9999
Temporary Codes	Q0000-Q0099
Diagnostic Radiology Services	R0000-R5999
Vision Services	V0000-V2999
Hearing Services	V5000-V5999

HCPCS Level III Codes

THE RANGE OF LOCAL LEVEL III CODES IS FROM W0000 - Z0000.

Local **Level III** codes are often used to describe:

➢ new procedures
➢ services or supplies
➢ procedures and services

NOTE: These local level III codes need to be obtained from your local Medicare intermediary.

Level III codes are also alphanumeric codes that start with a letter followed by four numbers.

A – Z (With 4 numbers following)

HCPCS Local Level III Codes & Modifiers

Local Level III codes are established and maintained by the local Medicare carrier in your area and will vary from state-to-state.

WHY SHOULD WE USE HCPCS?

➢ The use of **HCPCS** is mandated by HCFA for use on Medicare claims and is also required by most state Medicaid offices.

➢ **HCPC** codes improve a provider's ability to communicate services or supplies correctly without resorting to narrative reports.

➢ Their use reduces resubmission of claims for correction or review. If an inaccurate code is submitted, the claims' adjudicator must assign a code. That code, or its description, may be incorrect.

➢ Up-to-date and accurate **HCPC** codes on office routing slips allow office staff to assign fees quickly and efficiently to services and supplies, saving both time and money.

➢ Consistent submission of "clean claims" helps avoid an audit by a carrier due to frequent lack of specificity of claims.

➢ Use of **HCPC** is essential for accurate and complete reimbursement from Medicare. (Ex: an injection billed to Medicare with only a CPT code will not be reimbursed correctly. The drug administered must be identified with the correct Level II HCPCS code.)

➢ Supplies billed to Medicare as "*other than incidental to an office visit*" are not reimbursed unless identified with Level II HCPCS or Level III Local codes.

HCPCS MODIFIERS

A modifier is used to provide "*the means by which the health care professional can indicate that a service or procedure, that has been performed, has been altered by some specific circumstance*" but not changed in its definition or code.

HCPCS modifiers may be used to indicate the following:

➢ A service was supervised by an anesthesiologist

➢ A service was performed by a specific health care professional. (e.g. a clinical psychologist, clinical social worker, nurse practitioner, or physician assistant.)

➢ A service was provided as part of a specific government program

➢ A service was provided to a specific side of the body

➢ Equipment was purchased, rented or repaired

➢ Single or multiple patients were seen during nursing home visits

HCPCS LEVEL 1 MODIFIERS

The **HCPC** nationwide modifiers use a two-character alphabetic system. These modifiers may also be used to modify **HCPC Level I** (regular CPT) codes.

Some examples of the 1999 **HCPC** National Level II Modifiers are:

LT   Left side (used to identify procedures performed on the left side of the body)

RT   Right side (used to identify procedures performed on the right side of the body.

T1   Left foot, second digit

T2   Left foot, third digit

E1   Upper left, eyelid

E2   Lower left, eyelid

The list is extensive and found in the **HCPC** Coding book. Modifiers, similar to CPT codes are also added, deleted and modified each year. It is always best to check the book for the current modifiers.

An examples of using a **HCPC** National Level II modifier would be:

L8000 RT Breast prosthesis (RT indicating right side)

HCPCS Level III Modifiers

HCPCS are codes used by each regional Medicare fiscal intermediary. A Medicare fiscal intermediary is a large private insurance company that has been awarded the federal contract for processing claims by the federal government for a specific region. A Medicare fiscal intermediary may initiate the usage of a **HCPCS Level III** Modifier. That means using a **HCPCS Level III** modifier is regional carrier discretion and used only for the region that you are billing for.

Level III modifiers are also two alphanumeric modifiers beginning with the letters: **W, X, Y and Z**

Your local regional Medicare fiscal intermediary assigns the majority of these codes. A Medicare fiscal intermediary is an insurance company who won the bid for processing claims for government programs.

It is also important to note that **HCPCS National Level II** modifiers can be combined with CPT codes when reporting services to Medicare.

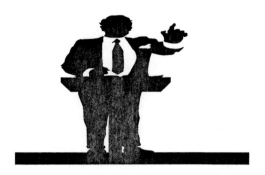

KEY POINTS REGARDING CPT AND HCPCS

CPT KEY POINTS

✓ All **CPT** codes are five digit numeric codes.

✓ **CPT** codes describe procedures, services and supplies.

✓ With few exceptions, **CPT** codes are accepted or required by all insurance carriers.

✓ **CPT** codes are self-definitive. With the exception of a few codes which contain the term SPECIFY in the description, each code has only one meaning.

✓ **CPT** codes are revised annually in December. Hundreds of **CPT** codes are added changed or deleted each year.

HCPCS KEY POINTS

✓ **HCPCS** codes are five-digit, alphanumeric codes. The first digit is a letter between A and Z and the second through fifth digits are numbers.

✓ The **HCPCS** coding system includes two-digit modifiers at the National and Local levels which may be alphabetic or alphanumeric.

✓ **HCPCS** codes describe supplies, materials, and services provided by medical professions.

✓ The **HCPCS** coding system is a three-level coding system consisting of CPT Level 1, National Level 2, and Local Level 3 codes.

✓ **HCPCS** codes are mandatory for billing Medicare carriers and some Medicaid carriers as well.

✓ **HCPCS** codes are revised annually in March.

✓ **HCPCS** codes follow a specific hierarchy of selection and use. **Local Level 3** takes precedence over **National Level 2** and **National Level 2** takes precedence over **CPT Level 1.**

✓ **HCPCS** coding can make a significant difference in your reimbursement from Medicare carriers.

✓ **CPT** and **HCPCS** coding can make a 25 percent difference in your reimbursement (plus or minus).

TRUE OR FALSE

1. T F   All **CPT** codes are five digit numeric codes.

2. T F   **CPT** books are divided into six sections.

3. T F   Modifiers are used with **CPT** and **HCPC codes** indicating a service/ procedure has bee altered.

4. T F   **HCPCS** includes codes for supplies, materials, injections, services not defined in the CPT book.

5. T F   **HCPCS** codes always start with a letter.

6. T F   The most common use for **HCPCS** codes is to bill Medicare for supplies, materials and injections.

7. T F   **HCPCS** codes are optional billing Medicare.

8. T F   **CPT** and **HCPCS** coding books should be purchased every year.

9. T F   Accurate **CPT** and **HCPCS** coding makes no difference in reimbursement.

10. T F   **HCPCS** Local Level 3 codes are assigned by your local Medicare intermediary.

11. T F   **CPT** codes have priority when reporting services provided to Medicare patients.

12. T F   **HCPCS** modifiers may be used with **CPT** codes.
(1-6, 8, 10, 12 True and 7,9, 11 False)

Claudia A. Yalden

CHAPTER 28

ICD-9 CM DIAGNOSTIC CODING

Since 1979, all coding of diagnoses on medical insurance claims in this country have been performed using the International Classification of Diseases (ICD-9 CM or ICD-9). The **ICD** system was established by the National Center for Health Statistics.

When the **ICD** system was established it meant submitted claims could be checked quickly by computer to ensure that payments are made only for those procedures that are considered medically necessary for the submitted diagnosis.

ICD-9 codes are updated annually. It is necessary to order a new coding book in September of each year. New codes go in effect October 1 but some Medicare carriers delay the reporting of new codes on provider office claims until January. Some of the commercial insurers do not accept the new codes until March 1.

ICD-9-CM codes are composed of codes with 3, 4 or 5 digits.

Codes with 3 digits are included in the **ICD-9-CM** as the heading of a category of codes that may be further subdivided by the use of a fourth and or fifth digit that provide greater specificity.

❑ A three-digit code is to be used **only** if it is not further subdivided.

❑ A fourth digit subcategorizes

❑ A fifth digit sub classifies

If further digits are provided, they must be assigned. A code is invalid if it has not been coded to the full number of digits required for that code.

You will need the ICD-9 book to fully understand what I am explaining. An example to look up would be:

ICD-9 Code 295. requires a 5th digit)

You first look up 295. and code it to the 4th digit.

Schizophrenia	295.9
> acute	295.8
> borderline	295.5
> disorganized	295.1

Then you will see the following 5th digit sub classification to be used with category 295.

0	unspecified
1	subchronic
2	chronic
3	subchronic with acute exacerbationk
4	chronic with acute exacerbation
5	in remission

What I have just shown you is how to look up a code.

Please remember that only a physician office can tell you what classification to use but this is something you should fully understand.

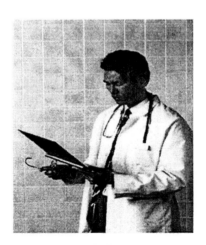

ICD-9-CM IS PUBLISHED IN THREE VOLUMES:

- **Volume 1** (Diseases Tabular/Numerical List) a numerical listing of diseases and injuries

- **Volume II** (Diseases Index) the alphabetical Index to Volume I Volume II is a three-part index to Volume I that includes three sections:

    > **Section 1** - The alphabetic index

    > **Section II** - Table of adverse effects to drugs and chemicals

    > **Section III** - The index to external causes (E Codes). This separate index is often forgotten; it will be help to mark it with a special tab as a reminder of its existence.

Volume III is used for reporting procedures rendered to inpatients. Volume III is included only in the hospital version of commercial ICD-9-CM books and is a combined alphabetical index and numerical index of inpatient procedures that is divided into three parts:

  Part 1 - Table List of Procedures by Anatomical Site

  Part II - Miscellaneous Diagnostic and Therapeutic Procedures

  Part III - Index to Procedures

Volumes I and II are used most commonly for coding diagnoses in the health care providers' offices and hospital outpatient departments.

Most medical publishing houses publish separate versions of ICD-9-CM for physician offices and hospitals. The Physician version has Volume I II combined in one book.

As stated, a health care provider generally does not use Volume III. They do use some additional codes created by HCFA to augment CPT codes on some Medicare claims. Again, these special HCFA codes are known as HCPCS Level II and III codes.

NOTE: Because most of the coding literature does not identify the coding system used when reporting code numbers, it is important to know the differences in the numerical codes for procedures. ICD-9-CM Volume III uses a two-digit main number augmented by two decimal digits for sub classification or procedures. CPT codes are a five-digit main. HCPCS Level II and III codes use a five character alphanumeric system.

CHAPTER 29

V CODES

V Codes - V Codes are to be used when there are factors influencing health status or valid medical reasons for contacting the health facility; but a definitive diagnosis or active symptoms ***cannot*** be stated. Diagnostic V codes main number is expressed as three character code which is the letter V and two digits with 4th and 5th digits added for a more descriptive description.

NOTE: **V codes** are used when 001-999 (the main part of the ICD) cannot record the "diagnosis" or "problems."

V Codes arise in three ways:

- When a person who is not sick encounters the health services for some specific purpose such as a donor of an organ or tissue to receive vaccination, to discuss a problem which is in itself not a disease or injury. It is more common among hospital out patients and patients of family practitioners.

- When a person with a known disease or injury encounters the health care system for a specific treatment of that disease or injury (e.g. dialysis for renal disease, chemotherapy, cast change.

- When some circumstance is present which influences the person's health status but is not in itself a current illness/injury. (e.g. personal history of certain diseases (diabetes, anemia, mental retardation) or a person with an artificial heart value in situ).

EXAMPLES ARE:

- Evaluation by cardiologist, internist, etc. prior to surgery when the patient has a history of heart problems.
- Removal of a cast applied by another physician
- Primary diagnostic codes for radiological and pathological procedures.
- Primary diagnostic code for rehabilitation and physical therapy procedures.
- Routine follow ups for possible recurrence of a tumor
- Well baby check ups.
- Annual physical examinations.

Examples are:

V10 Personal history of malignant neoplasm
  V10.0 Gastrointestinal tract
   History of condition
    V10.00 Gastrointestinal tract, unspecified

CHAPTER 30

E CODES

E CODES - External causes of injury and poisoning.

These codes describe the external cause of injury, poisoning or other adverse reaction affecting a patient's health. They are used to report:

- environmental events,
- industrial accidents,
- accidents occurring on a patient's own property,
- injuries inflicted by criminal activity,
- adverse effects of medicinal or biological substances,
- a condition occurring as sequalae 21 or more months after an injury.

These codes do not affect the increase or decrease of payment; however, they can expedite the processing of injury claims by indicating the injury is not reportable to a liability insurance program.

E Codes are secondary codes. The injury or poisoning is stated as the primary condition. There is a separate index for E codes. To locate the proper E code for an adverse reaction to a surgical or medical treatment, turn to the main term "Reaction" in the E code index.

Basic Guideline:

- The appropriate code or code(s) from 001.0 through V82.9 must be used to identify diagnosis, symptoms, conditions, problems, complaints, or other reason(s) for the encounter/visit.
- Documentation should describe the patient's condition, using terminology that includes specific diagnosis as well as symptoms, problems or reasons for the encounter.
- Codes 001.0 though 999.1 will frequently be used to describe the reason for the encounter.
- Codes that describe symptoms and signs as opposed to diagnosis, are acceptable for reporting purposes when an established diagnosis has not been diagnosed (confirmed) by the physician.
- Do not code diagnoses documented as "probable", suspected, questionable, or ruled out. Rather code the condition(s) to the highest degree of certainty for that encounter/visit such as symptoms, signs, abnormal test results, or other reasons for the visit.

   NOTE: This is contrary to the coding practices used by hospital and medical record departments for coding the diagnosis of hospital patients.

- Chronic diseases treated on an ongoing basis may be coded and reported as many times as the patient receives treatment and care for the condition(s).
- Code all documented conditions that coexist at the time of the encounter/visit and require or affect patient care treatment or management. Do not code conditions that were previously treated and no longer exist. However, history codes (V10-V19) may be used as secondary codes if the historical condition family history has an impact or current care or influences treatment.

CHAPTER 31

M CODES – HOSPITAL REPORT CODING ONLY

I am only mentioning M Codes because they are codes that are used in hospital billing only. I wanted you to be aware that they exist although you will never have to use them as a medical biller for a physician's office.

M Codes codes will appear in some hospital reports and should not appear on the physician's offices insurance claims.

The M appendix is very useful for the physician coder in deciding whether or not the Neoplasm Table should be used to locate the ICD-9 for a particular lesion.

The introduction to this appendix should be read carefully.

Most billing centers and physician's offices do not use the M Codes and you would be amazed at how many people do not even know about them.

CHAPTER 32

FORMS

➢ Superbill
➢ Explanation of Benefit
➢ HCFA 1500 Form

I have included a basic superbill. You will notice that the superbill has procedures and diagnostic codes listed. It also has a section for balance due. Some superbills have the fee listed next to the procedure.

The example Explanation of Benefits is from Blue Cross Blue Shield. Every insurance company has their own format and you will find they are all formatted differently but the information is all basically the same.

The HCFA Form is a HCFA 1500 form and the one that you will use for most insurance claims. It is always advisable to check with your state Medicaid office to find out if they use the standard HCFA 1500 form. The one state that has their own Medicaid form (called a D 9 Form) that I am aware of is Massachusetts Medicaid.

EXAMPLE OF A SUPERBILL

Casey Guido Medical Walk In Clinic
3 Medical Drive.
Billing City, New York 11777

Provider: _____
_____
_____

ID #: _____ Tax Id: _____

Name: _____
Address: _____
_____

Pat#: _____
Code: _____
Phone: _____

Document: _____
Date: _____
Time: _____

Code	Description	Code	Description
99201	Office Visit/Np/Level I	11730	Nail/Avulsion of plate
99202	Office visit/NP/Level II	11750	Excision of nail
99203	Office Visit/NP/Level III	11765	Nail excision
99204	Office visit/NP/Level IV	12002	Repair 2.6 cm to 7.5 cm
99205	Office outpatient visit new	17110	Destruction, Benign Lesion
99211	Office Visit/EP/Level 1	20550	Injection
99212	Office visit/EP/Level II	28080	Arthrotomy
99213	Office visit/EP/Level III	29580	Unna Boot
99214	Office visit/EP/Level IV	J1100	.
99215	Office outpatient visit est	99070	Custom Orthotics
99221	Initial hospital visit	29405	B-K Cast NWB
99222	Initial hospital care moder	29405A	B-K Cast NWB
99223	Initial hospital care high	99070	Custom Orthotics
99251	Hospital consult	99270	
99252	Inpatient/Hospital	93910B	PVD
99261	Hospital visit/Follow-up	93910D	Doppler Arterial Study
99262	Hospital visit/follow up	87070	Culture specimen for bacteri
99301	NP/Nursing home/Level I	078.10	Viral Warts - Unspecified
99302	NP/Nursing home/Level II	078.11	Condyloma Acuminatum
99302	NP/Nursing home/Level II	079.1	Echo Virus
99311	Evaluation & Mgmt	110.1	Dermatophytosis of Nail
99312	Evaluation & Mgmt	110.4	Dermatophytosis - of foot
99313	Followup nursing facility ca	170.8	M Neoplasm Short bones low
10060	Incision & drainage abscess	171.3	M.Neoplasm Soft tissue leg
10061	Incision complicated	250.0	Diabetes Mellitus w/o Compli
10120	Incision/removal foreign bod	250.00	Diabetes Mellitus - Type II
10121	I & D complicated	250.01	Diabetes Mellitus - Type I
10140	I & D of hematoma	250.02	Diabetes Mellitus - Type II
10160	Puncture aspiration abscess	250.03	Diabetes Mellitus.- Type I
11040	Excision/Debridement/skin	250.60	Diabetes w neuro manifest t
11041	Excision/Debridement/tissue	250.61	Diabetes w neuro manifest
11050	Paring of benign skin lesion	250.62	Diabetes w neuro manifest t
11051	Paring of 2-4 benign lesions	454.0	Varicose Veins/Lower Extremi
11420	Excision of Benign Lesion	680.7	Carbuncle of foot
11420	Excision Benign Lesion	681.11	Onychia and Paronychia of To
11421	Exc Benign Lesion(.06 - 10)	700.0	Corns and Callosities
11423	Exc Benign Lesion (2.1-3.0)	701.8	Hypertrophic atrophic skin N
11700	Nail Debridement manual		
11701	Nail Debridement		

Diagnosis: _____

	Family Aging Balances			Previous Balance	
Current	30	60	90	Today's Charges	
				Amount Paid	
				New Balance	

Remarks: _____
Next Appointment: _____

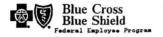 **Blue Cross Blue Shield** Federal Employee Program

Explanation of Benefits
THIS IS NOT A BILL

EXAMPLE OF AN EXPLANATION OF BENEFITS (EOB)

Blue Cross Blue Shield
3 Blue Way
Blue City, USA 800-123-4444

CLAIM NUMBER: 137880
DATE RECEIVED: 05/17/1999
DATE PROCESSED: 05/19/1999
DATE PAID: 05/20/1999
PATIENT NAME:
ID NUMBER:
PATIENT ACCT NO:

Patient: Papa Bear
           42 Berry Lane
           Berryville, New York 11777

SUMMARY OF STANDARD OPTION BENEFITS ON THIS CLAIM   BENEFIT CHECK SENT TO

PROVIDER NAME: SOUT   DATES OF SERVICE: 05/05/1999 - 05/05/1999

TYPE OF SERVICE	SUBMITTED CHARGES	NEGOTIATED SAVINGS	NONCOVERED CHARGES	EXP *	ALLOWABLE CHARGES	DEDUCT	COINS COPAY	OTHER COVERAGE	WHAT WE OWE	WHAT OW
OFF VISIT	45.00	11.00		610	34.00		12.00		22.00	1
TOTALS	$45.00	11.00			34.00		12.00		$22.00	$1.

* EXPLANATION OF CODES/REMARKS

610--THE COVERED CHARGES EXCEED THE ALLOWABLE CHARGES PROVIDED UNDER THE BLUE
CROSS AND BLUE SHIELD SERVICE BENEFIT PLAN FOR THESE SERVICES. COVERED
CHARGES ARE SUBMITTED CHARGES LESS ANY NONCOVERED CHARGES. BECAUSE THIS
PROVIDER IS A PREFERRED OR PARTICIPATING PROVIDER WITH THE LOCAL PLAN, YOU
ARE NOT RESPONSIBLE FOR THE DIFFERENCE BETWEEN THE COVERED CHARGES AND THE
ALLOWABLE CHARGES.

••

WHAT YOU OWE | SUMMARY OF OUT-OF-POCKET EXPENSES FOR 1999

			CALENDAR YEAR DEDUCTIBLE	CATASTROPHIC PROTECTION PPO	NON-PPO
CALENDAR YR DEDUCTIBLE	$				
PER ADMISSION DEDUCTIBLE	$				
COINSURANCE	$				
COPAYMENT	$	12.00	WHAT YOU HAVE PAID		
NON-COVERED CHARGES	$		INDIVIDUAL	$200.00	
RECERTIFICATION PENALTY	$		FAMILY	$303.63	$673	$673
			ANNUAL MAXIMUM		
TOTAL:	$	12.00	INDIVIDUAL	$200.00	
			FAMILY	$400.00	$2,000	$3,750

Any resubmission of eligible expenses on this claim must be received no later than December 31 of the calendar year
following the date of service or 90 days from the process date on this form, whichever is later.

EXAMPLE OF A HCFA FORM

PLEASE
DO NOT
STAPLE
IN THIS
AREA

PICA

HEALTH INSURANCE CLAIM FORM PICA

MEDICARE	MEDICAID	CHAMPUS	CHAMPVA	GROUP HEALTH PLAN	FECA BLK LUNG	OTHER	1a INSURED'S I.D. NUMBER	(FOR PROGRAM IN ITEM 1
(Medicare #)	(Medicaid #)	(Sponsor's SSN)	(VA File #)	(SSN or ID)	(SSN)	(ID)		

2 PATIENT'S NAME (Last Name, First Name, Middle Initial)

3 PATIENT'S BIRTH DATE MM DD YY SEX M☐ F☐

4 INSURED'S NAME (Last Name, First Name, Middle Initial)

5 PATIENT'S ADDRESS (No., Street)

6 PATIENT RELATIONSHIP TO INSURED Self☐ Spouse☐ Child☐ Other☐

7 INSURED'S ADDRESS (No., Street)

CITY   STATE

8 PATIENT STATUS Single☐ Married☐ Other☐

CITY   STATE

ZIP CODE   TELEPHONE (Include Area Code) ( )

Employed☐ Full-Time Student☐ Part-Time Student☐

ZIP CODE   TELEPHONE (INCLUDE AREA CODE) ( )

9 OTHER INSURED'S NAME (Last Name, First Name, Middle Initial)

10. IS PATIENT'S CONDITION RELATED TO

11 INSURED'S POLICY GROUP OR FECA NUMBER

a OTHER INSURED'S POLICY OR GROUP NUMBER

a. EMPLOYMENT? (CURRENT OR PREVIOUS) ☐ YES ☐ NO

a INSURED'S DATE OF BIRTH MM DD YY SEX M☐ F☐

b OTHER INSURED'S DATE OF BIRTH MM DD YY SEX M☐ F☐

b. AUTO ACCIDENT? ☐ YES ☐ NO PLACE (State)

b EMPLOYER'S NAME OR SCHOOL NAME

c EMPLOYER'S NAME OR SCHOOL NAME

c. OTHER ACCIDENT? ☐ YES ☐ NO

c INSURANCE PLAN NAME OR PROGRAM NAME

d INSURANCE PLAN NAME OR PROGRAM NAME

10d RESERVED FOR LOCAL USE

d IS THERE ANOTHER HEALTH BENEFIT PLAN? ☐ YES ☐ NO If yes, return to and complete item 9 a-d

READ BACK OF FORM BEFORE COMPLETING & SIGNING THIS FORM.

12 PATIENT'S OR AUTHORIZED PERSON'S SIGNATURE I authorize the release of any medical or other information necessary to process this claim. I also request payment of government benefits either to myself or to the party who accepts assignment below.

SIGNED   DATE

13 INSURED'S OR AUTHORIZED PERSON'S SIGNATURE I authorize payment of medical benefits to the undersigned physician or supplier for services described below.

SIGNED

14 DATE OF CURRENT MM DD YY ILLNESS (First symptom) OR INJURY (Accident) OR PREGNANCY(LMP)

15 IF PATIENT HAS HAD SAME OR SIMILAR ILLNESS GIVE FIRST DATE MM DD YY

16 DATES PATIENT UNABLE TO WORK IN CURRENT OCCUPATION MM DD YY   MM DD YY FROM   TO

17 NAME OF REFERRING PHYSICIAN OR OTHER SOURCE

17a I.D. NUMBER OF REFERRING PHYSICIAN

18 HOSPITALIZATION DATES RELATED TO CURRENT SERVICES MM DD YY   MM DD YY FROM   TO

19 RESERVED FOR LOCAL USE

20 OUTSIDE LAB? ☐ YES ☐ NO $ CHARGES

21 DIAGNOSIS OR NATURE OF ILLNESS OR INJURY (RELATE ITEMS 1,2,3 OR 4 TO ITEM 24E BY LINE)

1. ____   3. ____

22 MEDICAID RESUBMISSION CODE   ORIGINAL REF NO

23 PRIOR AUTHORIZATION NUMBER

24 A DATE(S) OF SERVICE From MM DD YY To MM DD YY	B Place of Service	C Type of Service	D PROCEDURES, SERVICES OR SUPPLIES (Explain Unusual Circumstances) CPT/HCPCS MODIFIER	E DIAGNOSIS CODE	F $ CHARGES	G DAYS OR UNITS	H EPSDT Family Plan	I EMG	J COB	K RESERVED FOR LOCAL USE

25 FEDERAL TAX I.D. NUMBER SSN EIN

26 PATIENT'S ACCOUNT NO

27 ACCEPT ASSIGNMENT? (For govt. claims, see back) ☐ YES ☐ NO

28 TOTAL CHARGE $

29 AMOUNT PAID $

30 BALANCE DUE $

31 SIGNATURE OF PHYSICIAN OR SUPPLIER INCLUDING DEGREES OR CREDENTIALS (I certify that the statements on the reverse apply to this bill and are made a part thereof.)

SIGNED   DATE

32 NAME AND ADDRESS OF FACILITY WHERE SERVICES WERE RENDERED (if other than home or office)

33 PHYSICIAN'S, SUPPLIER'S BILLING NAME, ADDRESS, ZIP CODE & PHONE #

PIN#   GRP#

(APPROVED BY AMA COUNCIL ON MEDICAL SERVICE 8/88) **PLEASE PRINT OR TYPE**

APPROVED OMB-0938-0008 FORM HCFA-1500 (12-90) FORM RRB-1500 APPROVED OMB 1215-0055 FORM OWCP-1500 APPROVED OMB 0720-0001-CHAMPUS

INSTRUCTIONS FOR FILLING OUT A HCFA 1500 FORM

Block 1A: Insured's Identification Number
Block 2:   Patients Name
Block 3:   Patient's Birth date and sex (use a 4 digit year format)
Block 4:   Name of Insured (no nicknames)
Block 5:   Patient's Address
Block 6:   Patient Relationship to insured
Block 7:   Insured's address
Block 8:   Patient status
Block 9:   Other Insured's Name (Enter "None" if patient has only a basic insurance plan and no supplemental policy.)
Block 10:   Patients Condition Related to
Block 10A: Employment - If condition is related to an on the job illness or injury a Workers Compensation claim should be filed.
Block 10B: Auto Accident (if yes write the appropriate two character state abbreviation where the accident occurred.)
Block 10C: Other Accident (means injuries that are reportable to a no-fault insurance program or liability insurance carrier.)
Block 10D: Reserved for Local Use (Enter the word attachment in this block if any additional information will be transmitted with this claim.)
Block 11-11C:Intended to cover a second primary insurance policy.
Block 12:   Authorization for Release of Information

Block 13:   Authorization for Payment of Benefits To the Provider
Block 14:   Date of First Illness, First Symptom, Injury, LMP (last menstrual period).
Block 15:   If patient has had same or similar illness give first date.
Block 16:   Dates Patient Unable to Work in Current Occupation
Block 17:   Name of Referring Physician or Other Source
Block 17A: ID Number of Referring Physician
Block 18:   Hospitalization
Block 19:   Reserved for local use
Block 20:   Outside Lab
Block 21:   Diagnosis or Nature of Illness or Injury
Block 22:   Medicaid Resubmission Code
Block 23:   Prior Authorization Number
Block 24A: Dates of Services
Block 24B: Place of Service
Block 24C: Type of Service
Block 24D: Procedures, Services, or Supply Codes
Block 24E: Diagnostic Code
Block 24F: Charges
Block 24G: Days or Units
Block 24H: EPSDT (Early and Periodic Screening for diagnosis and treatment). This is for certain Medicaid Programs. Check with your state.
Block 24I: EMG (Emergency Treatment). This is used for some managed care programs indicating a situation where you could not get prior authorization before the state of emergency treatment.

Block 24J: COB (Coordination of Benefits)
Block 24K: Reserved for local use (Leave blank unless
             instructed by a specific carrier to enter the
             carrier assigned Provider's Identification
             Number of the provider in a group practice.
Block 25:   Federal Tax ID Number
Block 26:   Patient Account Number
Block 27:   Accept Assignment
Block 28:   Total Charge
Block 29:   Amount Paid
Block 30:   Balance Due
Block 31:   Signature of Physician or Supplier
Block 32:   Name and Address of Facility Where
             Services Rendered

Common Errors

1. Typographical errors or incorrect information:

   - ✓ Procedure code invalid
   - ✓ Diagnostic code (missing 4th or 5th digit, code deleted, code does not match procedure code.
   - ✓ Policy Identification Numbers
   - ✓ Provider number
   - ✓ Total Amount Due On Claim
   - ✓ Incomplete or incorrect name of patient or policyholder
   - ✓ Treatment dates
   - ✓ Name and required UPIN, PIN, EIN or SSN missing
   - ✓ Referring physician identification number missing
   - ✓ Required prior authorization missing or incorrect

2. Attachments do not have patient and policy identification number on each page.

3. Staples or other defacement

4. EOB attached is not readable.

5. Failure to properly align HCFA form.

6. Signature missing

7. Procedure and diagnostic codes do not match.

CHAPTER 33

WEB ADDRESS PAGE

I have listed some web sites you might want to check out. Most of the sites will give you updated information concerning policy and HCFA changes. You may want to inquire about advertising with these organizations.

Use the search engines and search for Medicare, Medicaid and Blue Cross Blue Shield in your state.

- **Agency for Health Care Policy and Research**
  http://www.ahcpr.gov/

- **American Dental Association**
  http://www.ada.org

- **American Medical Association**
  http://www.ama-assn.org

- **Blue Cross Blue Shield Association**
  http://www.bluecares.com

- **Health Care Financing Administration (HCFA)**
  http://www.hcfa.gov

❑ **United States Department of Health & Human Services**
http://www.os.dhhs.gov

❑ **US Healthcare**
http://www.ushc.com

❑ **American Medical Womens Association (AMWA)**
http://www.amwa-doc.org/index.html

❑ **Podiatry Association**
http://www.biomech.com/specialties/podiatry

What Is The Academy Of Medical Billing?

The Academy of Medical Billing (AMB) is a subsidiary of CAY Medical Management (CAYMM). We are members of the Better Business Bureau. After reading Medical Billing The Bottom Line you will see that *anything is possible if you believe in yourself.*

I was once where you are now - searching, looking and investigating medical billing. Although I had experience in the field I didn't know the first thing about submitting a claim electronically, purchasing software and where to begin to have a home-based business.

In 1997 I formed the Academy to help other people and because of a growing need for qualified medical billers in the healthcare industry. Undoubtedly you have seen business opportunities available where you can purchase software and marketing training for exorbitant costs.

As experts in the industry, we have spoken to many people who have made the big investment; however, they still felt unqualified to market a service they did not understand. Their training did not include medical billing training, filing claims, or the proper usage of a surgical code, modifier, or how to get verification.

When you train with us you will be able to see first hand how a medical billing service and physician's office operates. You will be able to make phone calls to insurance carriers for eligibility verification and follow up on unpaid claims.

The Academy of Medical Billing is one of the country's first training Academy's that is also an actual medical billing center. We provide training in the comfort of your home, or at our medical billing office.

We want to help you succeed.
Your success is our success.
Let us help you visualize your goals.

800-221-0488

263

The Academy Of Medical Billing
Offers a Three Day Training Package

Offers a Three Day Training Package

$ 3,999.

Starting any business today requires capital. If you are really serious about owning and operating your own home-based medical billing business, then your time and money should first be invested in a solid training program.

Many colleges offer different courses about medical billing, however the individualized attention you receive from the Academy of Medical Billing is far superior and comprehensive.

Your success is dependent on our success. We want to see you succeed. We spend three fun filled days with you in the comfort of your home, hotel, or our office. The days are yours to ask questions and learn. We maintain a flexible time schedule to permit an in-depth learning environment.

Once we return to our own billing center you are not left as a number. We are there to support and guide you every step of the way. We cannot guarantee you a physician's office to bill for; however, we feel with the training you receive from us, your motivation and desire, success is only down the road.

Whether you take our training or not we wish you the best.

Go out there and do well!

What We Offer!

The Academy of Medical Billing (AMB) offers hands-on-individualized training. You work at your own pace and learn at a speed you are comfortable with. AMB realizes that new entrepreneurs entering the medical billing industry need more than marketing training. AMB offers medical billing and computer based instruction using MediSoft Advanced Patient Accounting Software. Graduates of AMB are confident and prepared to exercise their newly acquired knowledge with prospective clients when they leave AMB

What 2001 Will Bring Us?

Medical Billing is still the fastest growing home based business as we enter a new millennium. The reasons are obvious. The Clinton Administration was committed to eliminating paper claims. Yet, most doctors still send paper claims to the insurance company.

Electronic filing of claims is the future. It is presently costing a physician's office between $8. and $23. for each paper claim mailed. Billing centers can save practices thousands because they are not involved with high overhead, employee benefits, salaries, vacations, clearinghouse fee's, software updates, or maintenance fee's.

Why We Are Special?

All training is provided by an owner operated medical billing center and offers hands-on training. Claudia works in her office along with her staff when she is not training. Because of her success and the challenges Claudia faced, she realized that her experience could help others achieve their dream and not run into the problems she encountered.

Claudia feels that proper training is the foundation to success in the medical billing industry. Once your training is over . . . you are only a phone call away for continued support from AMB. AMB is striving to be the best training Academy in the country.

Includes

- Medical Billing The Bottom Line Revised Edition
- Identifying Your Prospects
- Marketing Workbook
- Sample letters and agreements
- Marketing Kit Samples

Topics to be discussed:

- Starting Out (phones, flyers, etc.)
- Finding Doctors
- Presentations
- Packets to mail
- Setting The Appointment
- Pricing Your Services – Three Ways!
- Agreements
- How A Physician's Office Operates
- Marketing With A Superbill
- Gathering Information To Complete A Claim Form
- Life Cycle Of A Paper Claim

Billing Service Video Training Seminar - Topics Covered are:

- Starting a business
- Writing a business plan
- Tools needed
- Overview of a doctor's office
- Organization of paper flow
- Overview of insurance billing
- Fees for Services
- Coding requirements
- Services offered
- Coding and charting
- Billing terminology
- Forms for data entry
- HCFA 1500 form
- Electronic Media Claims

At the end of the day we will help you write a press release and plan a strategic marketing plan.

Day Two - Let's Get Technical

Includes

- Understanding Medical Billing - A Step-by-step Guide
- Medical Billing Training Manual
- CPT and ICD-9 Coding Books

Day Two will be intense – but you will be on your way to gaining the confidence you need to succeed in the medical billing field.

We begin by covering the difference between CPT and ICD-9 codes. We go into HCPCS codes and Durable Medical Equipment.

You can finally visualize the making of a claim form.

In the afternoon you will spend a hands on day working from your medical billing training manual. It is with this information that will lead you to Day 3 – Inputting what you have learned and accomplished and applying it to the MediSoft Software.

Course Curriculum

- Types of health insurance
- Coordination of benefits
- Working with health insurance carriers and managed care.
- Collection of past due accounts
- Legal Considerations
- Billing procedures.
- Processing a paper insurance claim form
- Processing claims electronically.
- What is Durable Medical Equipment?
- What is a CMN?
- The Importance of Using HCPCS
- Wheelchair documentation
- Common errors with electronic billing
- Understanding an Explanation of Benefits
- Unpaid claims follow-up
- Glossary of Terms

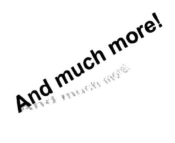

And much more!

Day Three - Let's Learn MediSoft
Day Three – Let's Learn MediSoft

Includes

- MediSoft Advanced Patient Accounting
- MediSoft Video Training Seminar
- MediSoft Manual
- Technical Training Manual

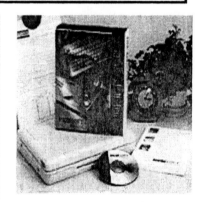

Day Three will be spent learning MediSoft Advanced Patient Accounting Software. You will be in front of the computer inputting the data you learned from the previous days. We will cover:

- Setting up a practice and setting up multiple practices
- Setting up patients
- Input patient data
- Input ICD-9 and CPT codes
- Set up insurance carriers
- Perform transaction entry
- Create claims
- Inputting Facilities

- Deposit entry
- Posting payments to a patients account.
- Different reporting features
- Format and Print a HCFA claim form
- Resubmission of a claim form

And Much more!

In addition - you will receive -

Claims Training Library -

Volume One - In the Getting Started section, learn why physicians need a billing service, how to establish your medical billing business, and how to market your services to healthcare professions.

Volume Two - The Guide to Health Insurance covers types of health insurance, coordination of benefits, working with health insurance carriers, and managed care.

Volume Three - The Billing and Collection section discusses collection of past due accounts, legal implications, credit policies, and billing procedures. In *How To Process Medical Claims* learn how to gather information to complete a claim, how to process a paper insurance claim form, and learn about the ease and value of processing claims electronically.

Billing Service Video Training Seminar -

- Starting a business
- Writing a business plan
- Tools needed
- Overview of a doctor's office
- Organization of paper flow
- Overview of insurance billing
- E and M coding requirements
- Services that can be offered

- Coding and charting
- Billing terminology
- Forms for data entry
- HCFA 1500 claim form
- Electronic Media Claims
- Fees for Services
- Sample letters and
  agreements

MediSoft Video Training -

MediSoft training classes are available on VHS video tape. With MediSoft training video tapes you get training on your own schedule, you can train new staff members immediately, and brushing up on specific operations is easy.

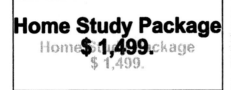
Home Study Package
$1,499.
Home Study Package
$ 1,499.

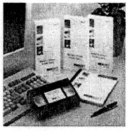

We are proud to offer the home study package for those who prefer to work at their own pace. The home study package includes:

- **MediSoft Advanced Patient Accounting Software**

- **MediSoft Video Help CD-ROM** - a tool to help you learn more about MediSoft and MediSoft Advanced Patient Accounting for Windows. This CD-ROM will walk you step-by-step through any function in MediSoft.

- **Claims Training Library** -

   Volume One - In the Getting Started section, learn why physicians need a billing service, how to establish your medical billing business, and how to market your services to healthcare professions.

   Volume Two - The Guide to Health Insurance covers types of health insurance, coordination of benefits, working with health insurance carriers, and managed care.

   Volume Three - The Billing and Collection section discusses collection of past due accounts, legal implications, credit policies, and billing procedures. In *How To Process Medical Claims* learn how to gather information to complete a claim, how to process a paper insurance claim form, and learn about the ease and value of processing claims electronically.

- **Billing Service Video Training Seminar** -

  - Starting a business
  - Writing a business plan
  - Tools needed
  - Overview of a doctor's office
  - Organization of paper flow
  - Overview of insurance billing
  - E and M coding requirements
  - Services that can be offered
  - Coding and charting
  - Billing terminology
  - Forms for data entry
  - HCFA 1500 claim form
  - Electronic Media Claims
  - Fees for Services
  - Sample letters and agreements

- **MediSoft Video Training -** MediSoft training classes are available on VHS video tape. With MediSoft training video tapes you get training on your own schedule, you can train new staff members immediately, and brushing up on specific operations is easy.

- **Technical Training Manual**

- **Listing of Providers In Your Area Who Do Not File Electronically**

$299. Package

MediSoft, the number one, most widely used medical billing software in the country. MediSoft is a windows based program and user friendly. You will receive all the necessary software to bill directly to National Data Corporation, the preferred MediSoft Clearinghouse.

Software support is provided by the technical department at MediSoft through their 800 number or on line. The Academy provides full medical billing and marketing support.

⇒ MediSoft Patient Accounting Medical Billing Software
⇒ MediSoft Software User Manual
⇒ Audio & Video Training Tutorial
⇒ Trouble Shooting Guide
⇒ Easy Quote Diskette & Guide
⇒ Marketing Book
⇒ Medical Billing Training Manual
⇒ Presentation Package

Minimum System
Requirements
486/66 processor
8 MB of RAM
Modem
Windows Operating System

WALL STREET JOURNAL – INSURERS MOVE TO CUT PILES OF PAPER WORK: *"Labor-intensive, error prone claims paper work is a major reason administrative costs gobble up, by some estimates, 20% or more of the health-care dollar."*

COMPUTERS IN HEALTHCARE MAGAZINE – *"About 80% of healthcare claims originate in the physician's office. 3 % of these claims are automated. The vast majority are still handled "manually." The potential savings from automating claims are significant by any measure, amounting to billions annually."*

HOME OFFICE COMPUTING MAGAZINE – MAKE BILLS YOUR BUSINESS: *"Medical billing primarily involves transmitting claims from doctors and dentists to insurance companies. Demand for medical billing centers, already strong, is expected to grow as pressure mounts to streamline the American healthcare system."*

HEALTHCARE FINANCIAL MANAGEMENT MAGAZINE – *"As the economy of sending claims electronically from providers (doctors) to payers (Medicare, Medicaid, and Insurers) becomes clear, growing numbers of payers seems to be moving away from paper claim forms."*

THE BEST HOME BUSINESSES FOR THE 90's – *(By work-at-home gurus Paul and Sarah Edwards). "Changes in the healthcare delivery system over the past few years have made doing medical billing one of the most desirable and accessible home-based businesses of the 90s."*

NEW BUSINESS OPPORTUNITIES MAGAZINE – *Rated Medical Claims Processing the 6th most desirable home-based business opportunity for the nineties stating, "There's a tremendous need for people to become involved in medical claims... The (health insurance) system is getting more and more complex...The market is unlimited."*